A Handbook on Drugs in Anaesthesia

Dr Pramod kumar
MD (BHU), FICA, QMAHO, FIAPM
Dean Medical Sciences TMU
Formerly Dean PDUMC Rajkot, GAIMS, RMCRCH

About the Author

The author Dr. Pramod Kumar has been a medical teacher in anaesthesiaology since 1975. He has been an ex faculty of IMS, BHD, MGIMS Wardha, SSSIHMS, Prasanthi Nilayam, MP Shah Medical College Jamnagar, PDU Medical College Rajkot & worked as Mdical Superintendent, Dean and Professor of Anaesthesia in eminent Medical Colleges of India. He is a founder member & President of Indian Society for study of Pain, Indian Society of Anaesthesiologists (ISA) – West Zone, Gujarat and Jamanagar branches. He has written more than 75 research papers in National and International journals and is a peer reviewer of IJA, Ind Pain, JACP and Asian Arch Anaesth, IJAA, IJCA. He has written several books e.g. Textbook of Anaesthesia, Textbook of Pain, Clinical Methods in Anaesthesia, MCQ in Anaesthesia, Guide to PNB, Terminal Cancer Care, Veterinary Anaesthesia, Anaesthesia in Dentistry, Pain in Cancer, CPR (in Gujarati) Atlas in PNB and coauthor in Pain Mechanisms and Pain Medicine and Year Book of Anaesthesia. He has received Life Time Achievement Award by ISSP I[st] SA-WZ, ISA Bhopal Award for Academic Excellence President Silver Medal ISSP and received seven oration awards. His Bio data is listed in American, International, Young Men and Women of achievement, Indo American and Indo European WHO's who.

About the Book - A Handbook on Drugs in Anaesthesia

This book "A Handbook of Drugs in Anaesthesia" has been written with an aim to provide the students of MD, DA, DNB, MD (Ay) Anaesthesiology a comprehensive, accurate and short account of drugs used in anaesthesa. This is relevant during theory and practical examination when going for viva voce for drugs. These topics have been dealt on a point to point basis providing a relevant account which is desirable in the examination. I hope this book will be helpful to the practitioners and students of Anaesthesia in examination and in practice. This further acts a ready reckoner for these topics.

Dr. Pramod Kumar
MD, DA, FICA, QMAHO

CONTENTS

1.	Mechanism of Action of Drugs	1
2.	Uptake and distribution of anaesthetic drugs	16
3.	Dorsal Horn Receptors	32
4.	Autonomic Nervous System	35
5.	Inhalational & Intravenous Anaesthetics	50
6.	Local Anaesthetics	80
7.	Non Steroidal Anti Inflammatory Drugs	96
8.	Opioids	101
9.	Opioids Drug Delivery	108
10.	Pharmacology of drugs used in cardiovascular system	117
11.	Respiratory and Adjuvant Drugs	134
12.	Central Nervous System	140
13.	Paediatric Drugs and doses	147
14.	Summary of drugs used in Anaesthesia	160
15.	Generic Drugs	169
16.	ASA Guidelines on labeling of pharmaceuticals for use in anesthesiology	172
17.	ASA Guidelines security of medications in the operating room	175
	Annexure 1: Mechanism of action of some drugs	177
	Annexure 2: Pharmacological Mnemonics	182

Chapter 1. Mechanisms of Action of Drugs

The initial doses selected and then titrating subsequent doses based on clinical response of the patient requires understanding of pharmacokinetic and pharmacodynamic principles. The former deals with drug concentration at site of action, while later explores the effect of drug concentration and its pharmacological effect involving cellular mechanisms of drug action, clinical evaluation of effects and variability in response.

Pharmacokinetics

Involves relationship between drug dose and plasma or effect site concentration, and is governed by absorption, distribution and clearance. There are various fundamental concepts governing the pharmacokinetics.

Volume of distribution

There is a dilution from high concentration of the drug injected to its diluted concentration in the plasma due to moving of drug in large volume. By knowing concentration in plasma, the volume can be measured.

Volume = amount (or dose) /concentration----------------- (1) or
Va (ss) = total drug / plasma concentration----------------- (2)
Concentration = amount / volume   -----------------(3)

However the volume of distribution of the drug depends on the properties of the drug.

A. Central volume of distribution

Reflects the volume of heart, great vessels, venous volume of upper and drug uptake by the lungs. The less lipophillic alfentanil results in less pulmonary uptake meaning less central volume for it than more lipophillic fentanyl or sufentanyl. So central volume reflects any metabolism that occurs between venous injection and the arterial sample. The mixing of bolus injection is not possible as the arterial drug concentrations are zero. Peak action comes between 30-40 s of the injection. This time is important determinant of anaesthetic induction. The time delay and recirculatory peaks have been shown in a mathematical model by Krejecle et al.(figure 1).

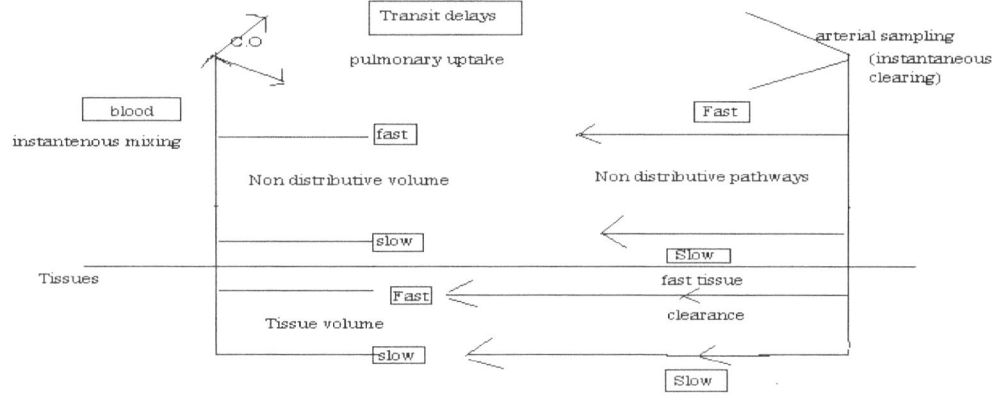

Fig.1: Mathematical model of volume of distribution

There are various factors affecting the central volume of distribution.
1. Arterial concentrations are higher initial concentration than venous sample.
2. Timing of the sample- over 2-3 minutes, the concentration of the drug falls rapidly. There is a higher value at 30 sec than the sample drawn at 5 min.
3. Total body water- in elderly the total body water decreases resulting in mitral reduced mixing volume leading to higher peak concentrations explaining the increased sensitivity in elderly patients to many drugs.

B. The peripheral volumes of distribution

In tissues represents additional volume attached to the central volume, by blood flow (inter compartmental clearance) the size of peripheral volume of distribution reflects the drug solubility in the tissue in relation to plasma. In spite of drugs constant physiochemical properties, the differences in body habitus and composition causes variation due to aging, increased body fat and decreased total water. Thus volume of distribution at steady state (Vdss) is a volume that relates the plasma drug concentration at steady state to the total amount of the drug in the body.

Clearance

The clearance is a process that removes the drug from a volume either by elimination or by transforming it into metabolites. The clearance is defined as the volume (measured as flow) that is cleared of drug per unit of time.

Hepatic clearance: Liver metabolizes drugs through oxidation and reduction (in cytochrome p-450 systems) hydrolysis and conjugation. The enzyme cytochrome p-450 can be induced by exposure to certain drugs or inhibited by drugs and diseases,. The conjugation and hydrolysis occur outside p-450 system. Conjugation transforms hydrophobic molecule into water-soluble ones by adding polar groups, which makes metabolites easier to excrete by kidney.[1]

The rate of metabolism for most of the drugs is proportional to the concentration of drugs flowing into the liver. The rate of drug flow into liver is liver blood flow (Q) times the concentration of drug flowing(C in flow). The rate at which drug flows out of the liver is Q times the concentration of drug flowing out (C outflow).

Thus the rate of hepatic metabolism by liver (R) is the difference between C inflow and C outflow times Q.

Rate of drug metabolism (R) = Q (C_{inflow} − $C_{outflow}$) --------------------4

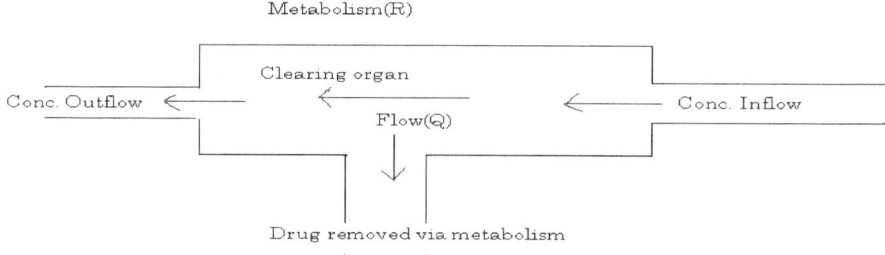

Fig2. Rate of drug metabolism

The rate of metabolism is also the clearance of the drug multiplied by the arterial concentrations.
Rate of drug metabolism (R) = Q (C_{inflow} − $C_{outflow}$) = C inflow X clearance—(5)

The clearance can be determined by dividing all the terms in equation 5 by the concentrations of the drug flowing into liver:

Clearance = rate of drug metabolism/ C_{inflow} = Q (C_{inflow}-$C_{outflow}$)/C_{inflow} ------(6)

The equation (6) now offers two definitions of clearance, each of which means:

Clearance = rate of drug metabolism/ C_{inflow} ----------------------(7)

The equation (7) means that clearance is proportionally constant that relates drug metabolism to the drug concentration. If liver is completely efficient then rate of drug metabolism will equal the rate at which drug is flowing into liver (Q X C_{inflow}), the rate of outflow (Q X $C_{outflow}$) will be zero and clearance will then equal hepatic blood flow (Q):

Clearance = Q [(C_{inflow} - $C_{outflow}$)/C_{inflow}] --------------------------------(8)

The above equation introduces the concept of extraction ratio, which the ratio between the amount of the drug flowing into the liver and the amount of the drug extracted (cleared).

The extraction (clearance) ratio (ER) = (Q (C_{inflow} – $C_{outflow}$)/ (C_{inflow}

Referring back to equation (7), the clearance equals the liver blood flow multiplied by the extraction ratio, Q X ER. Some drugs are flow dependent of their clearance. Any reduction in flow to liver reduces the clearance with high extraction ratio in a linear fashion. However the capacity of the liver to the metabolism flow dependent drugs vastly exceeds the usual flow of drug to the liver at typical clinical concentrations. Changes in hepatic function perceive will have little impact on the clearance of flow dependent drugs [2].

Any liver disease or changes in capacity due to enzyme induction will affect clearance of drugs like alfentanil having extraction ratio less than 1, where changes in blood flow will have little influence on the clearance as liver metabolizes only a fraction of the drug(Fig 3).

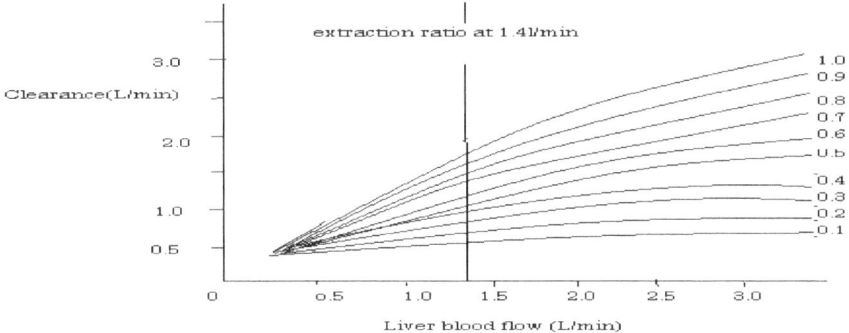

Fig 3 Changes in drug clearance as a function of liver blood flow with extraction ratios

The liver volume, blood flow and metabolic capacity decrease with advancing age. Hepatic enzymes can also be induced by other drugs or environment, smoking, increasing clearance of capacity limited drugs.

Renal clearance: Renal clearance of the drug from plasma is by glomerular filtration and direct transport into the tissues. Renal blood flow is inversely proportional with age as is the cretonne clearance, which can be predicted from the age X weight.

Creatinine clearance in man (ml/min) = 140 – age (yrs) X weight (kg)   -------(9)
                                                      >2 X serum concentration (mg%)

In women this concentration is 85% of the above value.

The equation 9 shows that age is an independent factor in creatinine clearance, which is decreased in old age, which applies to pancuronium. Above 85% of pancuronium is extracted by the kidney[5].

Tissue clearance: in some cases anaesthetic drugs are cleared in tissues e.g. blood, muscles and lungs as in case of remifentanyl which is cleared by nonspecific esterases located in muscles and intestines above as lungs, liver, kidney and blood contributes to its clearance.

Succinyl choline and mivacurium are metabolized in the blood by plasma cholin esterases about half of atracurium is metabolized in liver and rest half in plasma by Hoffman degradation. Later is a major route of metabolism for cis-atracurium which is unaffected by disease or genetic variations of cholinesterases. Tissue clearance can flow limited, capacity limited.

Distribution clearance

Drug can be removed temporarily from the plasma by the distribution clearance, which transfers the drug between plasma and peripheral tissues. It is the function of the tissue blood flow and the permeability of the capillary walls to the drug. Tissue blood flow varies non-linearly with cardiac output except in brain and heart. The permeability of vascular wall, tissue membrane is other component of tissue clearance. Permeability is function of lipophilicity. Propofol with high lipophilicity has a very high distribution clearance as it crosses the membrane rapidly while a highly hydrophilic glycopyrrolate is expected to have a slower distribution clearance because of difficulty in crossing membranes.

Protein binding

All anaesthetics bound to plasma proteins, which is governed by the law of mass action.

(Free drug conc.) of unbound protein binding sites ==== Bound drug----- (10)

K_{on} is rate constant for binding and K_{off} is rate constant for dissociation of bound drug from plasma proteins. At equilibrium the rate of K_{on}/K_{off} is solved fork.

$K = K_{on}$ = (Bound drug) _____(11)
K_{off} (free drug)(unbound protein binding sites)

There are more binding sites for anaesthetic drugs available. The unbound proteins sites can be reasonably approximated by n [protein], whereas protein is the plasma concentration of the binding protein and n is the number of binding sites for protein molecule. Since n is constant, it is included in our rate constant ; as dissociation rate constant Ka as.

Ka = (Bound drug)/(Free drug) --------------------------------(12)

If we define fu as free drug fraction of the drug

fu = (Free drug)/(Bound drug) + (Free drug) -------------------(13)

Combining the equations 12 and 13, the fu can be calculated in terms of unbound drug concentration

fu =1/Ka [Protein] +1   --------------------------(14)

The last equation shows that fraction bound to plasma protein depends on protein concentration alone and not on the drug concentration.The changes in protein binding also affect the clearance of drugs. Drug with high extraction ratio are removed from the liver (regardless of protein binding). Reverse change is seen with low hepatic extraction ratio drugs.

Stereochemistry

Most of the anaesthetics are racemic mixtures and the action of the enantiomers may not be identical. When a drug with a racemic mixture is injected; it is as if two drugs are given. However, drugs assays are usually insensitive to chirality. Thus concentration measured is actually a mixture of two separate drugs. The Pk and Pd of enantiomers of various drugs e.g. bupivacaine, mepivacaine and ketamine have been studied in the hope that d(+) isomer will provide the hypnosis and analgesia in associated with ketamine with its psychotomimetic effects. However there is little difference in therapeutic windows between stereo tactic racemic mixtures.

Genetics

Genetic difference in receptor structure refers to genetic diversity in drug metabolism. Later is due to a natural adaptive response of animals to an environment that can produce a huge variety of toxins. The enzyme diversity is maintained through natural selection to ensure survival and is evident with the drug therapy as unexpected toxicity, duration of action or lack of efficacy to administered drugs. Cytochrome P-450 2D6, also called debrisoquijne hydroxylase, seen in 7-10 of white population causes altered metabolism of the at least 40 drugs, one of those being codeine which produce no analgesia in these patients. Subjects with abnormal butyryl cholinesterase prolonged succinyl choline paralysis. Later effect is seen in Middle Eastern descent tribes. In India, particularly in saurashtra region, Bhanushali community has G-6-P-deficiency, which can interfere with metabolism of many drugs possibly including succinyl choline, which is avoided in these patients in G G Hospital, Jamnagar as a matter of protocol.

Pharmacokinetic models

Pharmacokinetics are classically represented by compartment models, such as the one-compartment model shown to the right. This model has a single volume and flow. The attraction of the one-compartment model is its simplicity. It is easy to visualize the body as a one-compartment model (particularly when it is wrapped in Spandex), into which we inject drug. The mathematics of the one compartment model are easy also. The initial loading dose to achieve a concentration is simply your target times V, the volume of the compartment. The infusion rate to maintain a target concentration is simply your target times Q, clearance.

If a human body was built like bucket, it would have a single volume and a single clearance. The math would be easy, but life would be dull. For all intravenous anesthetic drugs, it behave as if several buckets were connected together by pipes (figure 4- two compartment model and figure 5- three compartment model). The volume to the left in the two compartment model, and in the center of the three compartment model, is called the "central volume." The other volumes are called "peripheral volumes," and the sum of the all the volumes is the volume of distribution at steady state (or Vd_{ss}). The clearances leaving the central compartment for the outside is the "central" or "metabolic" clearance. The clearances between the central compartment and the peripheral compartments are called "inter-compartmental clearances."

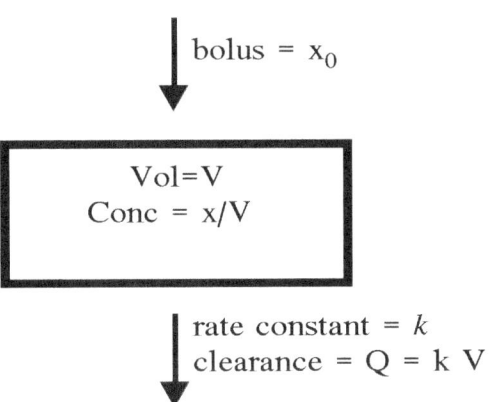

Figure 4: The one compartment model, with a single volume and flow term.

It is likely that the central (or "metabolic") clearance estimated by pharmacokinetic modeling has a true physiologic basis. It is also conceivable that the volume of distribution at steady state (Vd_{ss}) has a physiological basis: the partitioning of drug into all body structures at steady state.

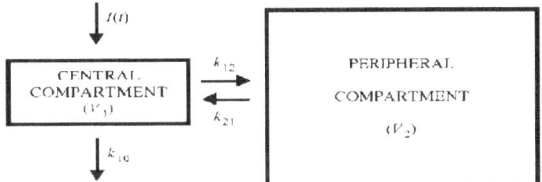

Figure 5: Two compartment pharmacokinetic model, with two volumes, (central and peripheral) and two clearances (central, and intercompartmental).

In three compartment models, it is speculated that the rapidly equilibrating volume (V₂) corresponds to vessel rich group and the slowly equilibrating volume (V₃) corresponds to the fat and vessel poor group. For highly lipophilic drugs in which a large V₃ may be explained by extensive distribution of the drug into fat. Mostly the volumes and clearances (except central clearance and Vd$_{ss}$) developed in pharmacokinetic models are simply mathematical constants derived from equations that describe the plasma drug concentrations over time. They are not direct measures of anatomic structures or human physiology.

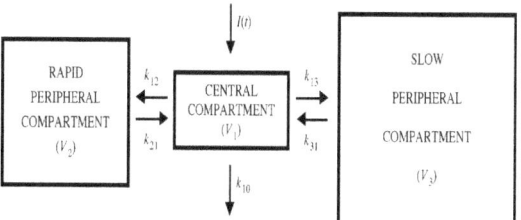

Figure 6: Three compartment model, with three volumes, (central, rapidly equilibrating peripheral and slowly equilibrating peripheral) and three clearances (central, rapid and slow intercompartmental).

The reason multicompartment models are used for the intravenous anesthetic drugs is that the plasma concentrations over time following a bolus of an intravenous drug resemble the curve in figure 7. For many drugs, three distinct phases can be distinguished. There is a rapid "distribution" phase (solid line) that begins immediately after the bolus injection. This phase is characterized by very rapid movement of the drug from the plasma to the rapidly equilibrating tissues. Often there is a slower second distribution phase (dashed line) that is characterized by movement of drug into more slowly equilibrating tissues, and return of drug to the plasma from the most rapidly equilibrating tissues (i.e, those that reached equilibrium with the plasma during phase 1). The terminal phase

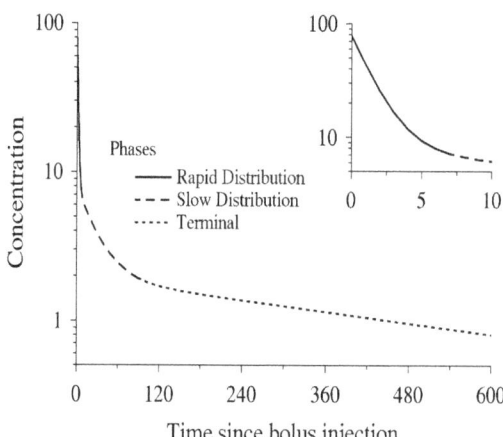

Figure 7: Shape of curve following intravenous bolus injection.

(dotted line) is a straight line when plotted on a semi-logarithmic graph. The terminal phase is often called the "elimination phase" because the primary mechanism for decreasing drug concentration during the terminal phase is drug elimination from the body. The distinguishing characteristic of the terminal elimination phase is that the relative proportion of drug in the plasma and peripheral volumes of distribution remains constant. During this "terminal phase" drug returns from the rapid and slow distribution volumes to the plasma, and is permanently removed from the plasma by metabolism or renal excretion.

Curves which continuously decrease over time, with a continuously increasing slope (i.e., curves that look like figure 5), can be described by a sum of exponentials. In pharmacokinetics, one way of notating this sum of exponentials is to say that the plasma concentration over time is:

$$C(t) = Ae^{-\alpha t} + Be^{-\beta t} + Ce^{-\gamma t} \qquad \text{Equation 1}$$

where t is the time since the bolus, C(t) is the drug concentration following a bolus dose, and A, α, B, β, C, and γ are parameters of a pharmacokinetic model.

Equation 1 in modeling pharmacokinetics describes the data. In particular, one can use it to describe both the onset and offset of drug effect. The "classic" method of describing the offset of drug effect is to use the terminal half-life. This is not a good idea for drugs described by multicompartmental pharmacokinetics, because the half-life relates only to 1 parameter, γ, while all 6 parameters in equation 1 influence the rate of offset of drug effect.

Time course of drug effect

There is a time lag between plasma drug concentration and effect site drug concentration. The time course of drug effect lags about a few minutes behind the rise in arterial concentration (hysteresis). The plasma concentration peaks at the moment the infusion is stopped, leading to a decrease in concentration. However the drug action still continues despite this decrease. The rapid blood brain equilibration reduces the hysteresis.

The relationship between the plasma k the site of drug effect is modeled with an effect site model (fig 10). The site of drug effect is connected to the plasma by a first order process, as described earlier. The equation, which relates effect site concentration to plasma concentration, is;

$$dC_e/dt = K_{e0}C_p - k_{e0}C_e \text{---------------}(43)$$

where C_e is the effect site concentration, C_p is the plasma concentration; K_{e0} is the rate constant for elimination of drug from the effect site. It is more easily understood in terms of the reciprocal, $0.693/K_{e0}$. the half time for equilibration between the plasma and the site of drug effects.

The constant K_{e0} has a large influence on the rate of rise of drug effect, the rate of offset of drug effect and the dose that is required to produce the desired drug effect. In conclusion, the pharmacokinetics involves fundamental physiologic process e.g. metabolism, protein binding, tissue distribution and drug transport to the site of drug effect. Pharmacokinetic models are mathematical showing relationship between doses & concentration, help in determining how best to give drugs to achieve a therapeutic objective, but only when this relationship is truly understood, these can be applied in understanding clinical onset of drug effect.

Pharmacodynamics

Pharmacodynamics describe the relationship between drug concentration and pharmacological effects. This involves transduction of biological signals, clinical evaluation of drug effects and biologic availability.

Transduction of biologic signals 'Receptor theory'

A receptor is a component of a cell that interacts selectively with an extra cellular compound to initiate a biochemical change, a cascade of alterations that represent observed effects of the drug. The binding of drug to a receptor determines the quantitative relation between dose and effects, its selectivity and explains the pharmacological activity of agonists, antagonists & inverse agonists. The receptor is a mediator or amplifier of the drug on the biologic system.

Classific receptor

The concept of receptor is attributed to Paul Erlich (1854-1915) who observed that a drug couldn't act unless they are bound. The binding of a ligand (drug molecule) to its receptor or follows the laws of chemical reactions (analogous to Michael's mentor enzyme) kinetics and summarized by the following

$$[L] + [R] ==== [LR]$$

where k_{on} the rate constant for the ligand binding to the receptor, k_{off} is the rate constant for the ligand dissociating from the receptor, [L] is concentration [R] is the concentration of the unbound receptor. Since k_{on} are units of [L] multiplied by the units of [R] over time, typically the unit of k_{off} are units of [LR] over time. The term dissociation constant Kd.

The term Kd or dissociation constant defines characteristics of ligand/receptor in detection at equilibrium

$$K_d = \frac{[L][R]}{[LR]} = \frac{K_{off}}{K_{on}}$$

When enough drug is administered to occupy 50% of the receptors the measured Kd is directly equal to the drug concentration. The reciprocal of is Ka (association constant) is its protein binding and is a measure of the affinity of the drug for the receptor for the receptor. Hence a drug with low Kd constant has a high Ka, thus high affinity for the receptor.

In practice it is difficult to measure precise drug receptor occupancy as if the drug receptor complex is an intermediate step in the production of a specific effect. An effect can me any biochemical or physiological variable that is measurable by an altered biochemical compound, an enzyme level, a physiological variable e.g. heart rate and blood pressure or a response to any graded input in the biological system e.g. response to a nerve stimulator in case of a muscle relaxant.

The delivery of a drug to a given receptor is time and dose dependent. For central compartment receptors there is instantaneous equilibrium after intravenous injection. For other routes there is a delayed onset of the response to the drug, occurring anywhere in the path between drug receptor binding and clinical effect. This is seen in drug receptor complex induced secondary messenger changes, increased enzyme synthesis and time required for physiological changes (e.g. reduced fluid content)

Receptor agonists and antagonists

Agonist drugs induce an effect mimicking endogenous hormones or neurotransmitters, when bound to a receptor. This effect may be stimulatory or inhibitory. The term affinity in relation to antagonist is a measure of attraction between the drug and receptor. A drug with low affinity does not bind to the receptor while that with a high affinity produce the effect at a lower dose.

Full agonists completely activate a receptor while partial agonist does it only partially (fig 8). The difference is due to differing intrinsic activity of each drug. The drugs with some affinity for a receptor may produce different levels of activation for the receptor, thus named full or partial agonists, related to the ability of the drug to stabilize the high affinity state of the receptor.

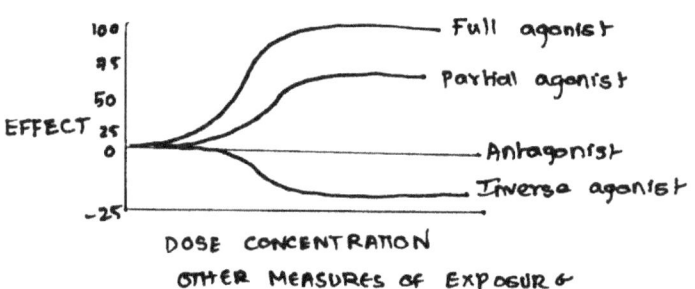

Fig. 8. Effect of various ligands on receptor responses. (Full agonist- just less than 100 Neutral agonist – no activity, Inverse agonist – super antagonist)

Antagonists inhibitor or prevent receptor mediated effect by competing for receptor occupancy and can be replaced by a large concentration of the agonist, permitting agonist to produce the expected effect. However, a non competitive antagonist binds irreversibly to the receptor complex, with a permanent loss of effect clinically vecuronium is a competitive antagonist of acetyl cholinesterase inhibitor which prevent acetyl choline breakdown and raises later concentration and replaces vecuronium.

Inverse agonists are called super- angtagonists as they decrease receptor response below the baseline. EEG response to R019=4063 is a example of reverse antagonist.

Inactive or activated receptor states

Interaction between ligand and receptor follows the law of mass action according to classic receptor theory. There may be an interaction at the molecular level initiating a change in receptor conformation, changing it from inactive (R) to an activated state(R*) proteins. (Guanine nucleotide (G) proteins or second messengers (effectos, E) which initiates a cascade of cellular responses. The agonists cause spontaneous conversion from R to R* (Fig 10) or stabilize the receptor site R* while inverse agonists stabilize R whereas neutral antagonist bind equally to R and R*. Once the agonist bind to R* this complex activate second messenger pathway and removed from the equation. Conversely the inverse agonist drives the equal on to the left, stabilizing the R configuration.

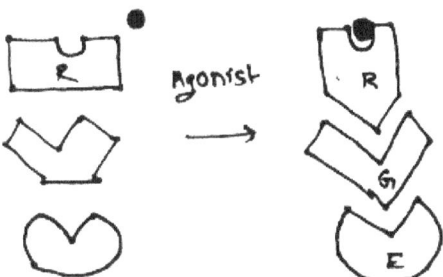

Fig.9. classific receptor activation from inactive (R) to activated state(R*) which then interacts with G and then E

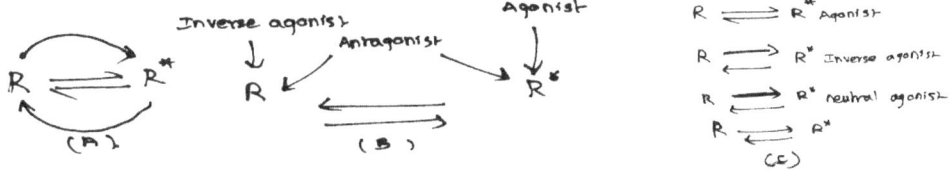

This response often varies from less than baseline to a true zero response level. Because antagonists are neutral (by definition) they bind equally R and R* presently agonist response with changing the equilibrium between R and R* hence do not change

Fig10. Spontaneous conversion of inactive R to active R*

The baseline response. Many classic antagonists are in truth inverse agonists, rather than neutral antagonists. The inverse agonists may be useful in seizures and congestive heart failure

Receptor structure

Receptors are located in many places in the cell outer cell membrane, cytoplasm, intracellular organelle membranes and nucleus. The overall physical structure of receptor depends on the type of receptor considered as well as its location. The cytoplasmic receptors bind to ligands that travel lipid layers to reach cytoplasm or nucleus e.g. steroid and thyroid hormone receptors. In anaesthesia excitable cell membrane portions eg. Membrane receptors, ligand gated, and voltage gated ion channels (Fig11)

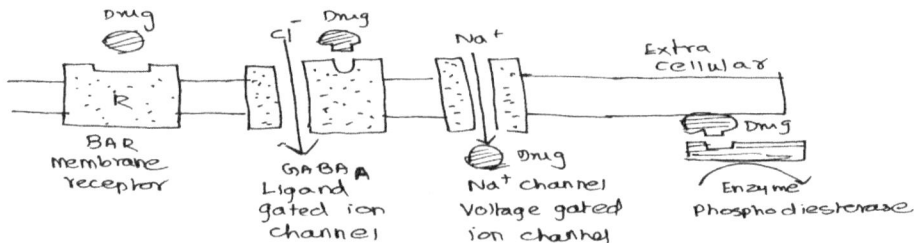

Fig11. Four types membrane associated inhibitory targets-Membrane G protein, Ligand gated, Voltage gated, and enzyme mediated many endogenous hormones and exogenous drugs are water-soluble so unable to access lipid layers. So they bind to extracellular membrane via coupling to second messenger via intermediate proteins or via a larger ion channel complex.

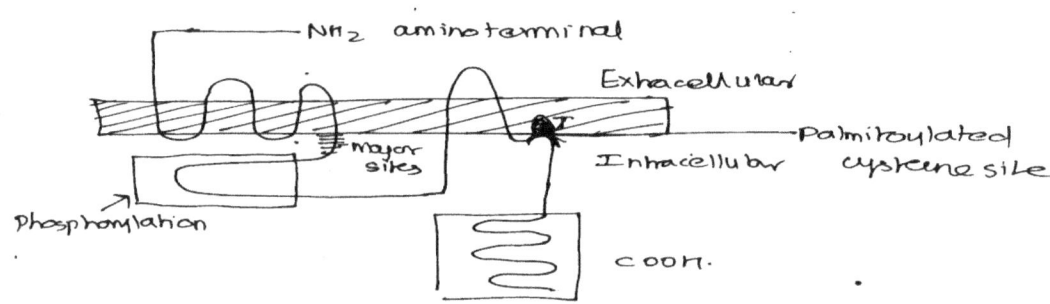

Fig 12. G coupled protein receptor with seven membrane domain, an NH_2 terminal, intracellular COOH terminal three extracellular and four intracellular loops, g protein Major sites and phosporylated sites in third loop.

Guanine nucleotide (G) protein coupled receptors

This is one of the most common methods by which membrane receptors translate agonist occupancy into intracellular action. They are most abundant and reveal an extracellular amino terminus containing an extracellular amino terminal, a carboxyl terminal, a fatty acid palmitoyl cysteine site, three extracellular and four intracellular loops. Major sites of G protein interaction are in 3rd and 4th intracellular loops while major site for phosphorylation.

The amino acid sites are hydrophobic so act counter to water soluble hormone. Here the structure activity relationship is critical, as chemical structure of a drug must match the 3 dimensional configuration of the binding area of a receptor. A subtle change in drug structure may dramatically alter the ability of the drug to bind to specific receptor[11] (Fig 13)

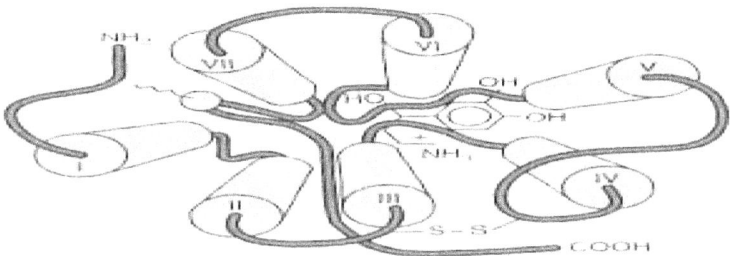

Fig.13. Schematic of three dimensional structure of adrenergic receptor (a prototype G-protein coupled receptor)

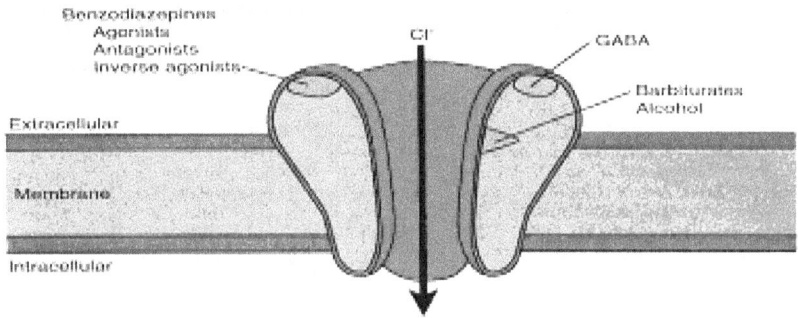

Fig. 14. Schematic of GABA- benzodiazepine complex(a prototype of ligand gated ion channel complex)

Ion channels

The ion channels mediate neutral signaling by modulating ion permeability in the electrically excitable membrane. These are Na+ channels, which are voltage dependent, in the presence of a voltage sensor. During depolarization these charges are more outward causing configuration changes and rearrangement of ion pairs, resulting in sodium permeability. Blockade of Na+ channels by local analgesics is one of the examples of pain insensibility.

In addition there are ligand gated ion channels e.g. nicotine acetyl choline and $GABA_A$ receptors the combination of a classic receptor protein plus an ion channel results in a ligand gated ion channel, having both hydrophobic and control charged transmembrane regions of the former two receptors. The binding at ligand gated channel complex, enhances or dampen an already existing ion flux, e.g $GABA_A$ site binding of benzodiazepines, barbiturate and alcohols facilitating endogenous GABA leading to increased inhibitory chloride ion flux in the CNS.[11,12] (Fig14)

Second messengers

After binding to receptor there are a series of rapid biochemical events called second messengers. Many membrane receptors couple to their primary second messengers via G protein which require energy in the form of GTP. There is triggering of effector cascade by stimulating (GS, Gq) and inhibitory (G1G0)
G proteins and the physiological effects depends on specific G protein and subsequent cellular response. G proteins have three sub units α, β and γ. While α subunit confers specificity, the later two stimulate second messengers and anchor regular kinases to the cell membrane, leading to enhanced phosphorylation.

Then there are other second messenger systems like adenyl cyclase playing a part in glucagons and histamine, phosphatidylinositol system playing a part in α_1 adrenergic, endothelin and muscarinic (M1, M3, M5) agonists. Stimulation of receptor and second messengers lead physiologic effects in a given tissue depending upon receptor, G protein and second messengers.

Molecular pharmacology

Molecular biology techniques provide a unique opportunity to study receptors and their structure at DNA level. It has lead to a discovery of many receptors and more receptor subtypes. Future drugs will target receptor and its subtype. All proteins are encoded in human genomes as nucleic acids. every amino acid present in a protein is encoded, so if DNA sequence of that encodes a particular receptor protein, is determined, then the primary structure of the receptor can be deduced. These fragments of DNA (genes) can be inserted with special cells that will express (manufacture, assemble, and deliver to appropriate location in the cell) receptor protein in high quantity. This can help in studies of receptor itself, involve potential discovery of new receptors and receptor subtypes and finally new investigational changes can be rapidly screened for effects on various receptors.

Molecular biology now includes creation and study of whole animals (usually mice) with altered physiological features using transgenic and knock out technology, with or without a specific gene respectively. Novel functions for specific adrenergic receptor subtypes (Eg. Role of α and β in mediating vasoconstriction and $\alpha 2$ in sedation and CNS mediated hypotension have been discovered.

Clinical evaluation of drug effects

After a physiological effect is produced it can be evaluated clinically by dose response curves, efficacy, potency and median effective dose (ED_{50}), the median lethal dose (LD_{50}) and the therapeutic effect.

1.) Dose response curve- the dose response relationship is time independent relationship between dose, concentration (X axis) and the measured effects. The measured effect can be an absolute response (Twitch height) a normalized response (% twitch height decrease) or a population response (fraction of subjects moving at incision). The standard equation for this relationship is the hill equation:

$$\text{Effect} = E_0 + (E_{max} - E_o) \frac{C^y}{C^y_{50}+C^x}$$

Where E_0 is baseline effect in the absence of drug, E_{max} is the maximum possible drug effect. C is concentration, C_{50} is concentration associated with 50% of peak drug effect (potency). Exponent Y relates to sigmoid, city and steepness of the curve. If Y = 1 and curve is plotted on a standard X-axis, than the curve appears to hyperbolic. If Y is greater than 1, then curve is sigmoidal (Fig 15) if X axis is plotted on a log scale, the curve will be sigmoidal, regardless of the value of Y.

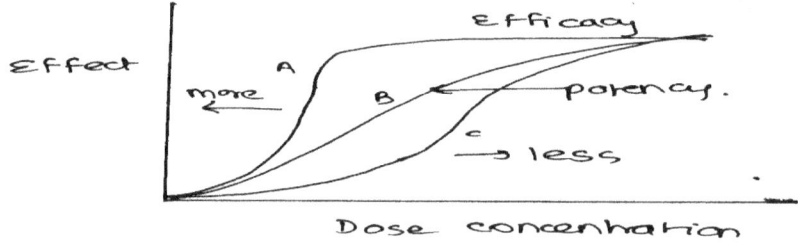

Fig 15. Dose response curve

Effect of agonist and antagonist on dose response curve

The dose-response curve is modified by agonist and antagonists. For two agonists with identical affinity (Ka) for a given receptor and identical second messenger coupling, the identical affinity (Ka) for a given receptor and identical second messenger coupling, the resultant dose response curve should be superimposable in case, otherwise it is parallel With rightward shifted curve for drug with lower affinity. If two drugs are administered simultaneously, then the linear relationship expected is not seen e.g. neuromuscular transmission measured change in effect on twitch height is not linear when receptor occupancy declines from 100 to 90 % as compared with change from 80 to 70 % occupancy.

The maximal response to full agonists and less than maximal response to partial agonists at the same receptor occupancy, may be due to the ability of full agonist to stabilize R* most effectively. Finally, addition of a competitive antagonist shifts the dose response curve to the right (higher agonist concentration is required to achieve effect) this dose response curve generated by the addition of antagonist in the presence of a non competitive fails to demonstrate attainment of maximal response at any dose because blockade of effect (antagonism) cannot be reversed.

Effective dose and lethal dose

The ED_{50} is the dose of a drug required to produce a specific effect in 50% of the individuals to whom it is administered. The LD_{50} is the dose of a drug required to produce death in 50% of patient (animals) to whom it is administered. The therapeutic index of a drug is the ratio between LD_{50} and ED_{50} (LD_{50}/ED_{50}). Hence the higher the therapeutic index of a drug, the safer the drug is for clinical administration because LD_{50} is far higher than the ED_{50} (Fig 16)

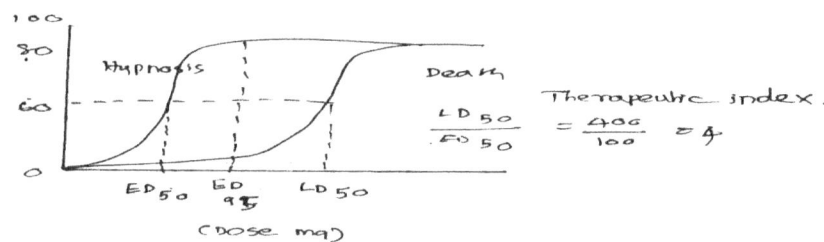

Fig16. Relationship between ED_{50} and LD_{50} and therapeutic index

Efficacy and potency

Efficacy is a measure of intrinsic ability of a drug to produce a given physiologic or clinical effect. Efficacy is influenced by receptor coupling to G protein, activation of second messengers, and the ability to generate ultimate physiologic responses. The scale to describe intrinsic efficacy at a given receptor varies from 0 to 1. The efficacy for full agonists is 1.0 for neutral antagonists it is zero which varying between 0 to 1 for a partial agonist.

Potency refers to the quantity of drug that must be administered to produce specific effect, two drugs may have same efficacy but if one drug produces the maximum effect only at 1 mg while the second produces the maximum effect at 100 mg then the second drug is less potent. (Fig 17)

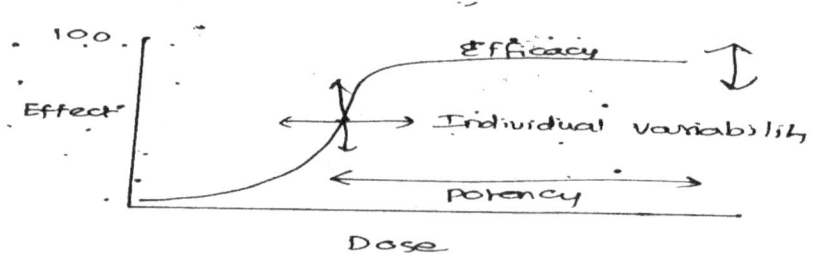

Fig 17. Relationship between efficacy, potency and individual variations related to dose response curve

Desensitization

It is broadly defined as waning of physiologic responsiveness to a drug over time. In perioperative period acute desensitization of vasodilatation response to nitroprusside occurs, therefore it is necessary to increase concentration over time. The stimulation of receptor pathways result in activation of kinases (G protein) that phosphorylate specific regions of the receptor, thus preventing further interaction of the receptor with G proteins and/or second messengers. Thus desensitization provide a negative feedback mechanism to receptor stimulation. Effectively desensitization shifts the dose response curve to the right (Fig 8) curves B or C compared with curve and/ or decreases maximal drug effect, hence both efficacy and potency decrease. Desensitization is a feature of many diseases in elderly e/. g. Congestive heart failure, hypertension and diabetes, when hormone (agonist) concentration is elevated. Thus cautious doses are utilized in such patients.

Increased receptor sensitivity

It is the opposite of desensitization. Long-term exposure to a drug often results in compensatory responses by the receptor system, by increasing receptor number (density). If receptor antagonist is suddenly discontinued, continuing β adrenergic blockers during perioperative period. Abrupt discontinuation leaves the myocardium vulnerable to exaggerated heart rate and ionotropic response to tracheal intubation.

Biologic variability

Individual variation in response to an identical dose of a drug occurs due to difference in absorption, distribution, metabolism and excretion of the drug. An identical number of molecules present at the effector site produce different responses in different patients. The relationship between patient variability and a typical dose response curve is shown in in addition to desensitization, factors that effect pharmacodymanic responses include age, genetic variability and concurrent diseases.

Age- many drugs with CNS effects (benzodiazepines, opioids, propofol) appear to be intrinsically more potent in the elderly, the requiring lower concentrations.

Genetic variability

If a receptor or second messenger is defective or hyperactive, then pharmacodynamic alterations in the drug effect will be noted. Malignant hyperthermia manifested in 1:20,000 anaesthetics given, is triggered by halothane and a hypermetabolic response results. It is related to abnormal calcium release and uptake by sarcoplasmic reticulum.

Disease states

Various diseases result in decreased perfusion e.g. in heart failure, or decreased perfusion as in renal failure. Diabetes, thyroid diseases, adrenal diseases, myasthenia gravis and hypertension alter receptor function. It can lead to desensitization, there is other function elimination clinically muscle relaxant doses are reduced in such patients.

References

1. Krejcie TC, Arrane MJ, Gentry WB et al. A recirculatory model of the pulmonary uptake and pharmacokinetics of lidocaine based on analysis of arterial and mixed venous blood data from dogs. J Pharmacokinet. Br opharan 1997;25:169.
2. Shafer S. principals of pharmacokinetics and pharmacodynamics. In: Long Necker DE, Tinker JH, Morgan GE (eds). Principals and practice of anaesthesiology. 2nd edition. ST Louis, Mosby year book, 1997, 1159.
3. Wilkinson GR, Shand DG. Commentary: A physiological approach to hepatic drug clearance. Clin pharmacol. 1975, 18:377.
4. Danzlger RS, Tobin TD, Becker LC et al. The agea associated decline in glomerular filtration in healthy normotensive volunteers: lack of relationship to cardiovascular performance. J Am Geriatric society, 1990; 38:1127.
5. Upton RA, Nguyen Th, Miller RD et al. Renal and biliary elimination of vecuronium (ORG NC 45) and pancuronium in rats. Anaesth analg, 1982;61:313-6.
6. Davis D, Grossman SH, Kitchell BB et al. The effect of age and smoking on the plasma protein binding of lignocaine and diazepam. Br J Clin Pharmacol, 1985;19:261-5.
7. Perssom J, Hasselstrom J, Maurset A et al. Pharmacokinetics and non-analgesic effects of S- and R- ketamines in healthy volunteers with normal and reduced metabolic capacity. Eur J Clin Pharmacol 2002, 57:259.
8. Scatt JC, Ponganis KV, Stanski DR. EEG quantification of narcotic effect: The comparative pharmacodynamics of fentanyl and alfentanil. Anaesthesiology, 1985;62:234.
9. M Stapel feldt WH. The autonomic nervous system. IN : Schwinn DA (ed): scientific principals of anaesthesia. Vol 2, Philadelphia, current medicine, 1998.
10. Berkowitz DE. Cellular signal transduction. In: Schwinn DA (ed). Scientific principals of anaesthesia. Vol 2. Philadelphia, current medicine, 1998.
11. Firestone L, Quinlan J, Gyulai F. mechanisms of anaesthetic action. In Schwinn DA (ed). Scientific principals of Anesthesia, Vol 2, Philadelphia. Current medicine 1998.

CHAPTER 2. Uptake and Distribution of Inhalational Agents

Basis of Uptake and Distribution

The anaesthetic brain concentrations are developed and sustained without excessive depression till surgery lasts and a rapid recovery is needed. The knowledge of factors governing relationship between the delivered and brain (or heart or muscle) concentration is essential for an optimum anaesthesia.

Inspired to Alveolar Anaesthetic Pressures

The alveolar partial pressure governs partial pressures of anaesthetic in all body tissues, which then later should ultimately equal it. The partial pressure of inspired anaesthetic can be controlled precisely by high inflow rates of the delivery system.

Effect of Ventilation

Rate of rise of alveolar anaesthetic concentration (F_A) rises towards the concentration being inspired (F_I) and alveolar ventilation. After preoxygenation, the un- opposed effect of ventilation rapidly increases the alveolar concentration ($F_A/F_I = 1$). A 95% level of oxygen occurs in 2 minutes when a high flow system is used (Fig. 4.1). However, the solubility of anaesthetics is higher than O_2 and N_2, which leads to larger transfer of anaesthetic to the blood, through lung. This uptake opposes the effect of ventilation to increase alveolar concentration. At low inspired concentration the F_A/F_I ratio is determined by the balance between the delivery (through ventilation) and its removal by uptake. If uptake removes 1/3 of inspired anaesthetic, the F_A/F_I equals 2/3 and vice versa.

Factors Effecting Uptake

A. Factors raising the alveolar concentration, assuming a constant inspired anesthetic concentration, and no uptake by blood:

1. The inspired concentration (FI). The rate of rise is directly proportional to the inspired concentration.
2. The alveolar ventilation (Valveolar)
    a. The larger the minute alveolar ventilation (Valveolar), more rapid the rise in alveolar concentration (FA).
    b. Inspired gas is diluted by the FRC, so the larger the FRC, as a fraction of Valveolar, the slower the alveolar rise in anesthetic concentration.
    c. For ventilatory rates over 4 breaths, the ventilatory rate does not make any difference at the same Valveolar.
3. The time constant (TC)

The time required for flow through a container to equal the capacity of the container. If 10 liter box is initially filled with oxygen and 5 l/min of nitrogen flow into box then TC is volume (capacity)/flow.

TC = 10 / 5 = 2 minutes.

So, the nitrogen concentration at end of 2 minutes is 63%.

The time constant for the lungs is FRC/Valveolar.

Time Constant % washin/washout
1	63%
2	86%
3	95%
4	98%

The time constant for the anesthesia circuit is circuit capacity/FGF.
4. The larger the FRC, the slower the washin of a new gas.
5. The rate of rise of the alveolar concentration (FA/FI) is greatly slowed by anesthetic uptake by the blood.

Factors that Increase or Decrease the Rate of Rise of FA/FI

Increase
Low blood solubility
Low cardiac output
High minute ventilation
High pulmonary arterial to venous partial venous partial

Decrease
High blood solubility
High cardiac output
Low minute ventilation
Low pulmonary arterial to venous partial venous partial

B. Factors determining uptake by blood.
1. Solubility in blood:
   a. The blood/gas partition coefficient.
   b. The relative capacity per unit volume of two solvents (e.g. gas and blood) to hold the anesthetic gas.(ie. blood-gas partition coefficient of 1.4 means that each milliliter of blood holds 1.4 times as much isoflurane as a milliliter of alveolar gas does).
   c. The relative molar amount in equal volumes of blood and gas when the partial pressures are equal.
   d. Other things equal, the more soluble the anesthetic, the more drug will be taken up by the blood, and the slower the rise in alveolar concentration.

Table 1 : Partition coefficients at room temperature

Anaesthetic	Blood gas	Brain blood	Liver blood	Kidney blood	Muscle blood	Fat blood
Desflurane	0.45	1.3	1.4	10	2.0	27
Nitrous oxide	0.47	1.1	0.8	-	1.2	2.3
Sevoflurane	0.65	1.7	1.8	1.2	3.1	48
Isoflurane	1.4	1.6	1.8	1.2	2.9	45
Enflurane	1.8	1.4	2.1	-	1.7	36
Halothane	2.5	1.9	1.2	-	3.4	51
Diethyl ether	12	2.0	0.9	0.9	1.3	0.5
Methoxyflurane	15	1.4	0.9	0.9	1.6	38

2. Cardiac Output:
   a. The flow of blood through the lungs determines the amount of blood available to remove anesthetic gas.
   b. The greater the cardiac output, the slower the rise in alveolar concentration.
   c. Mathematically, changes in cardiac output have exactly the same influence on anesthetic uptake from the lungs as changes in solubility, since both influence exactly the same process: the size of the storage capacity of the blood for anesthetic agent over a given time interval.

3. The mixed venous anesthetic concentration:
   a. The higher the mixed venous concentration, the slower the anesthetic uptake.
   b. Initially 0.
   c. At equilibrium, the venous partial pressure = arterial partial pressure = alveolar partial pressure (e.g. uptake = 0).

d. The uptake from the lung, in liters of gas/minute:
e. The rate of rise of the mixed venous concentration depends on the tissue uptake of the anesthetic.

4. Tissue uptake of anesthetic:
    a. The tissue uptake (including blood) equals the uptake from the lungs.
    b. The same factors which govern uptake by the blood from the lungs govern uptake by the tissues from the blood:
        1. The tissue/blood partition coefficient (tissue solubility)
        2. The tissue blood flow.
        3. The tissue anesthetic concentration (analogous to the mixed venous tissue concentration).
    c. Tissue uptake, in liters of gas/minute =
    d. The rate of rise in tissue anesthetic concentration is proportional to tissue blood flow.
    e. The rate of rise in tissue anesthetic concentration is inversely proportional to the tissue capacity.
        1. The tissue capacity is: tissue volume x tissue solubility
    f. Just as discussed for the lungs, the tissues have a time constant:
1. time constant = solubility x volume / flow.
2. The fat governs the uptake of all anesthetics, until equilibrium is reached.
   g. The contribution of each tissue to the mixed venous partial pressure is the tissue anesthetic partial pressure * the flow to that tissue.
   h. The body can be roughly divided into 4 tissue groups, vessel rich group (brain, heart, lungs, kidney, splanchnic bed, glands), the muscle group, the fat group, and the vessel poor group (bones, cartilage, ligaments):

Group	% MASS	%CO
VRG	10	75
MG	50	18
FG	20	5.5
VPG	20	1.5

C. Unifying the above concepts:
1. Wash in of gas to the FRC occurs very fast (within 1 minute), so we will ignore it.
2. The alveolar/inspired partial pressure ratio approaches 1 with time.
3. V xF U - 1 = FF alveolar inspired Lung inspired alveolar

    Where ULung = uptake from lung and is the rate of drug delivery to the lungs, inspired alveolar FxV while ULung = B x Q x ((PA-Pvenous)
Barometric pressure
(Blood-gas solubility (λ), cardiac output (Q), and alveolar-to-venous partial pressure difference (PA - Pv)) is the rate of drug leaving the lung.

D. Metabolism
a. About 10-20% of halothane is eliminated through metabolism. This May be related to halothane hepatotoxicity.
b. About 2.5% of enflurane is metabolized.
c. No significant metabolism of isoflurane, nitrous oxide, or desflurane.
d. Sevoflurane is broken down into Compound A by CO_2 absorbants (baralyme and soda lime). Compound A is nephrotoxic in large doses. Most studies to date suggest that this is NOT a clinical issue with sevoflurane, even at low flow.

In case of enflurane, isoflurane or halothane which are moderately soluble, are compensated by a high concentration and to offset slow induction. The induction with 5% halothane is as rapid as induction with 8% sevoflurane, despite a fourfold solubility of halothane[2].

Mapelson Hydraulic Model (intuitive model)

A. The model consists of 5 upright cylinders.
1. The cylinders represent the inspired reservoir (mouth), the alveolar gas, vessel rich group, the muscle group, and the fat group.
2. The arrangement of the cylinders is as follows :(Fig 1)
3. The cross sectional surface of each cylinder corresponds to its capacity (volume * tissue solubility).
4. The four peripheral cylinders are connected to the alveolar gas cylinder by pipes at their bases. The diameter of the pipes correlates to the blood/gas partition coefficient times the cardiac output to each group, (except for the connection between the inspired reservoir (mouth), where the diameter of the pipe represents alveolar ventilation.)
5. The height of the column of fluid in each cylinder corresponds to the partial pressure of the anesthetic in that cylinder.

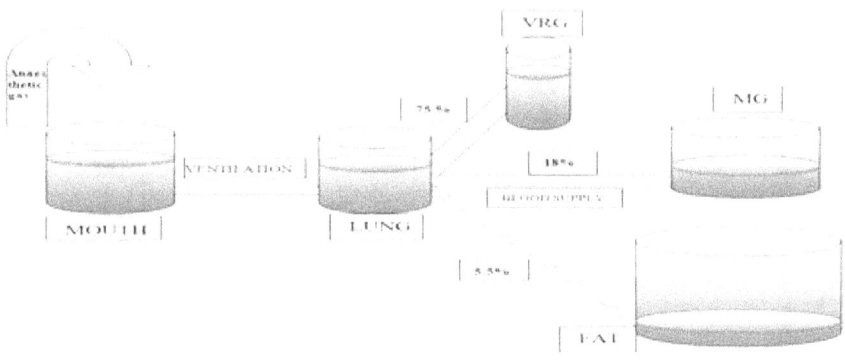

- The cross sectional surface of each cylinder corresponds to its capacity (volume * tissue solubility)
- The diameter of the pipes correlates to the blood gas partition coefficient times the cardiac output to each group
- The height of the column of fluid in each cylinder corresponds to the partial pressure of the anesthetic in that cylinder

Fig.1. Mapleson Hydraulic Model

B. Mapleson's analogy for inhaled anaesthetics of varying solubility:
1. The cross-sectional area of the vessels must be proportional, not only to the volume of the tissues but also to the solubility of the anaesthetic concerned in the tissues.
2. If two anaesthetics of different solubility are to be represented, two versions of model are needed.
3. For a low solubility anaesthetic (Fig 2 A).

1. All the compartments are small
2. The pipes are represented as small because the low solubility of anaesthetic is less carried by given blood flow

3. To achieve equilibrium for least soluble of anaesthetic small quantity of anaesthetic has to go in to the system.
4. For a high solubility anaesthetic (Fig 2 B) All the compartments are large. The pipes are represented as larger because the high solubility of anaesthetic is more carried by given blood flow To achieve equilibrium for high solubility of anaesthetic large quantity of anaesthetic has to go in to the system through the same sized ventilation pipe and therefore it takes longer time.

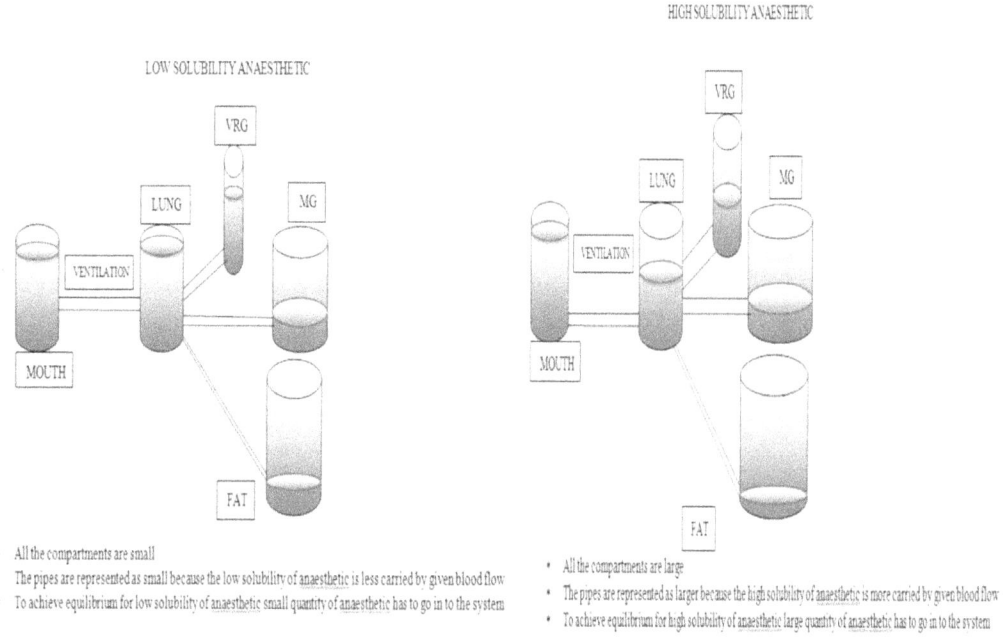

Fig 2. Mapleson Analogy for A. Low and B. High solubility Anaesthetics

The Concentration Effect

The inspired anaesthetic concentration also influences the alveolar concentration and the rate of attainment of that concentration[5]. At a 100% inspired concentration the rate of rise is very rapid and uptake no longer limits F_A/F_I levels. At 100% inspired concentration the uptake creates a void drawing the gas down the trachea, replacing the gas taken up. Due to 100% concentration of replacement gas, uptake cannot modify the alveolar concentration. This explains the more rapid rise of N_2O than the rise of desflurane despite their identical blood/gas partition coefficient.

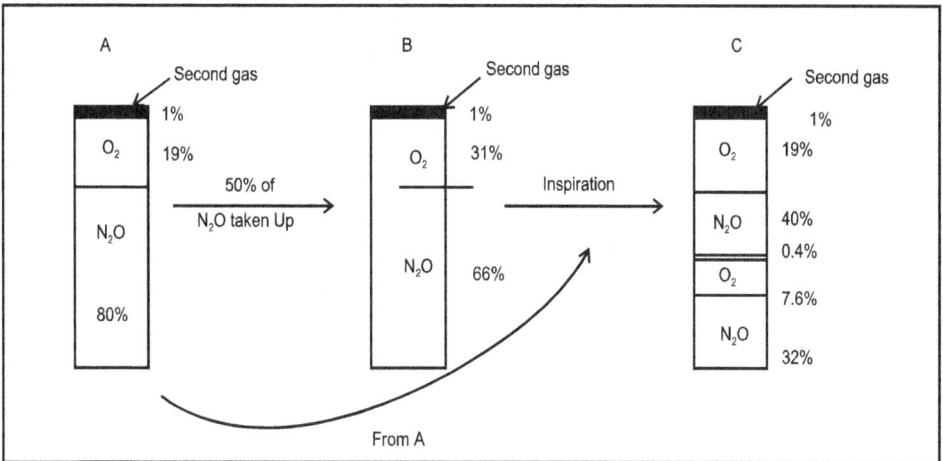

Fig 3 : The concentration effect. A. Lung filled by 80% N_2O and 19% O_2. uptake does not halve the N_2O concentration but the second gas is increased. Restoration of lung volume by same concentration as A increases N_2O concentration and second gas.

The contraction effect results from concentrating effect and increase in inspired ventilation[6] (Fig. 3). First rectangle represents a lung containing 80% N_2O. If half of this gas is taken up, residual 40% volume exists in a total of 60 volume, yielding a concentration of 66.7%. Thus uptake of ½ of the N_2O does not halve the concentration, because remaining gases are concentrated in a smaller volume, created by a void of uptake. If this void is filled up, the final concentration equals 72%.

This explanation is too simplistic as it ignores some effects of ventilation[7]. In controlled ventilation with volume control, the augmentation in inspired concentration is limited to the period of expiratory pause. This limitation is minimized in spontaneous ventilation.

The impact of the concentration effect on F_A/F_I may be thought of as identical to the impact of change of solubility[8]. As the inspired concentration increases, the effective solubility decreases as seen in case of N_2O at 1% inspired concentration.

Second Gas Effect

The factors that govern the concentration affect also influence the concentration of any gas given concomitantly[9]. The second gas applies to halothane or isoflurane when administered with N_2O. The loss of volume due to uptake of N_2O, concentrates the halothane. The replacement taken up by increased ventilation benefits the latter.

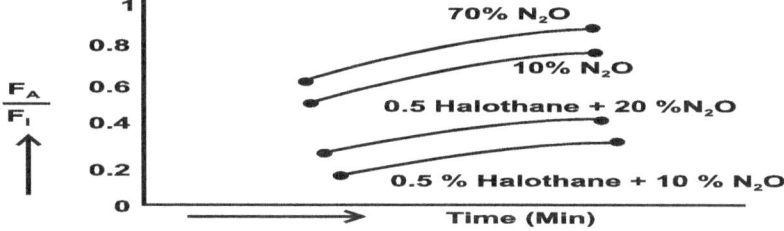

Fig. : Second gas effect

Both the concentration and the second gas effects were demonstrated in dogs, who received 0.5% halothane in 10% and 70% N_2O. The F_A/F_I for N_2O rose rapidly with 70% N_2O (Fig 4) similarly F_A/F_I for halothane rose more rapidly when 70% N_2O was inspired than that with 70% (Second gas effect).

Percutaneous Loss

The anaesthetic drug may be lost by transcutaneous movement, transvisceral movement and metabolism. The transcutaneous movement is small[10]. The loss of N_2O per alveolar anaesthetic (N_2O) equals 5 to 10 mL/mt with 70% alveolar concentration. There are more losses through viscera and plasma during surgery which are usually small relative to total uptake[11].

Metabolism of Anaesthetic

The loss of anaesthetic drug by biodegradation is significant. There is a 50% biodegradation of halothane and 75% of methoxyflurane when taken up[12]. Halothane decays more rapidly on recovery from anaesthesia than isoflurane due to its less solubility in blood[13]. Secondly, the anaesthetizing concentrations saturate the enzyme responsible for its metabolism.

Inter-tissue Diffusion

Carpenter et al[13], examined the washin and washout of isoflurane, enflurane, halothane and methoxyflurane given simultaneously for fixed periods of time. Analysis suggest a 5 compartmental model for all the drugs. The half-times for four of these compartments were consistently related to washin and washout of the lungs, VRG, muscle group and fat group. However, an additional compartment with a half-time of 300 minutes (between muscle and fat) accounted for 1/3 of the drug taken-up by diffusion of anaesthetic form lean tissue to an adjacent thin layer of fat, e.g., pericardial fat, perirenal fat and subcutaneous fat.

Factors Modifying the Rate of Rise of F_A/F_I

The factors governing the rate of delivery to lungs and its removal from lungs alter the alveolar concentrations of anaesthetics are ventilation and circulation along with drug solubility.

Effect of Ventilation

By increasing delivery of anaesthetic to the lungs on increased ventilation accelerates the rise of F_A/F_I[1] (Fig. 5). A change in ventilation produces a greater change in F_A/F_I with more soluble anaesthetics (ether), which triples the ether concentration in 10 minutes. In case of halothane it doubles, while scarcely affecting N_2O concentrations. Effect of solubility observed in poorly soluble N_2O, the rate of rise is rapid even with hypoventilation. With soluble agents e.g., ether, most of it is taken up, so uptake double with increased volumes of ventilation. Any change from spontaneous to controlled ventilation produces greater effect with more soluble agents, needing a caution.

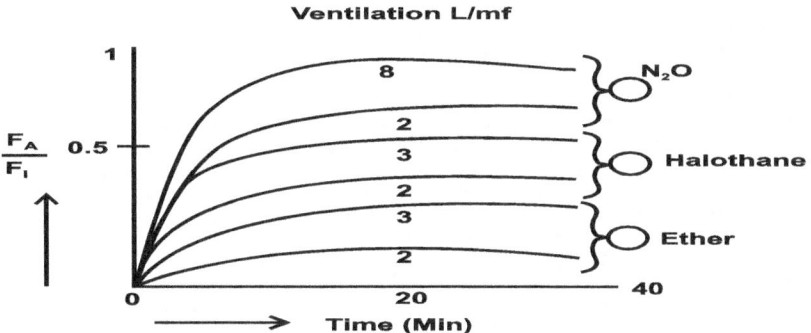

Fig. 5 : F_A/F_I rises rapidly with ventilation, solubility modifies the effect of ventilation

Anaesthetics themselves may alter ventilation and uptake[3] e.g., desflurane, halothane, isoflurane and sevoflurane which are profound respiratory depressants, decreasing anaesthetic delivery to the alveoli[3]. Doubling the inspired concentration does not alter the alveolar concentration at a given time, producing little absolute changes. Anaesthetics can exert a negative feedback on their own alveolar concentration during spontaneous ventilation and their safety.

Cardiac Output

In the previous, discussion cardiac output was assumed to be constant. An increase in cardiac output augments uptake and hinders the rise of F_A/F_I[14]. The cardiac output scarcely affects alveolar concentration of a poorly soluble agent while influencing the concentration in alveoli of a soluble agent(Fig. 6). This effect is similar to that seen in ventilation. There is no effect on F_A/F_I ratio in poorly soluble agent N_2O, while in case of a soluble agent the rate of rise is rapid at any cardiac output, nearly all of the drug is taken up and a halving of blood flow through lungs must concentrate arterial partial pressure (doubling it).

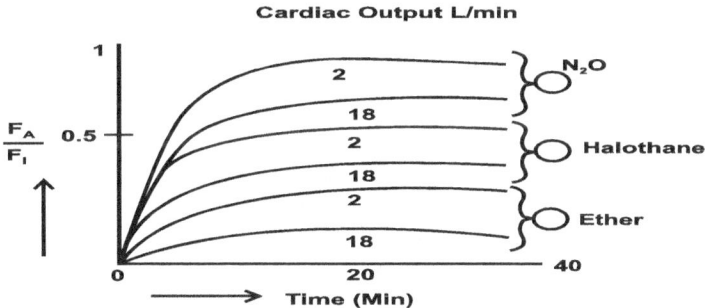

Fig.6 : Effect of cardiac output in alveolar drug concentration.

This effect of solubility is visible in case of shock when high alveolar concentrations are produced in case of a soluble agent. So, a caution will reduce further depression of circulation. In shock there is an increase in ventilation and a decrease in cardiac output. So, nitrous oxide is more reliably used in shock as compared to halothane. Later may themselves depress cardiac output. In contrast to ventilation, there is a positive feedback in this case. Depression decreases uptake, increases alveolar concentration and this in turn further decreases uptake and accelerates the rise of F_A/F_I[3], specially if the agent is soluble. This requires a caution with halothane and enflurane, in shock specially with controlled ventilation.

Ventilation Perfusion Changes

The concomitant changes in ventilation and perfusion should ideally produce no change when uptake is the term used all along. The alveolar to venous partial pressure difference if increased due to cardiac output and ventilation reduces their impact on uptake, thus a proportional rise in the rate of F_A/F_I. The magnitude of rise in F_A/F_I depends on distribution of the increased output. If increase is distributed to all tissues, the increase is very small[15], as in hyperthermia and thyrotoxicosis. However, if this increased perfusion is diverted to VRG, a rapid equilibration occurs and VRG soon has the partial pressure equal to, when it left lungs, so, cannot remove more anaesthetic from lungs. So after a few minutes increase in ventilation is not matched, by a slight increase in uptake now, leading to a rapid rise in F_A/F_I. The children with high VRG show a faster rise in F_A/F_I, leading to faster and intense anaesthesia[16], further compounded by a high perfusion of brain.

Ventilation Perfusion Ratio

Till now alveolar and arterial pressures were taken to be equal as seen in normal patients. Considerable decrease in arterial partial pressures occurs with emphysema, atelectasis and congenital heart disease. This produce an increase in alveolar end-tidal partial pressures and decreases the arterial anaesthetic partial pressures. The solubility of anaesthetic cause a relative change, poorly soluble agents increasing end-tidal concentration while reducing arterial partial pressure. The opposite occurs with a highly soluble agent[17].

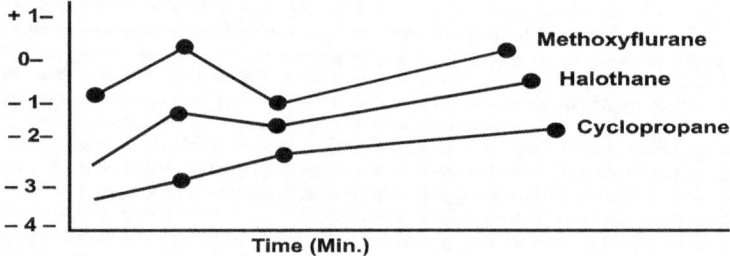

Fig.7: Rise of methoxyflurane normal, while reduced with cyclopropane in right lung ventilation.

The ventilation perfusion ratio abnormality increases ventilation relative to perfusion in some alveoli while reverse occurs in other alveoli. The poorly soluble agents are not found to observe a parallel changes in increased ventilation and alveolar and arterial anaesthetic partial pressure in these alveoli. When ventilation decreases relatively to perfusion as in atelectatic segment there is no additional anaesthetic when the later mixes with normal segment blood the mixture contains less arterial partial pressure of the drug. In case of highly soluble agents, the anaesthetic partial pressure rises to a higher level when coming from an alveoli receiving more ventilation than perfusion. (Fig. 5). This increase in anaesthetic compensates for the lack of anaesthetic taken up in the atelectatic segment. These effects are shown in Figure 7, where cyclopropane, a poorly soluble agent does not have compensatory mechanism as compared to a soluble agent methoxyflurane, where partial pressures are hardly changed. An intermediate effect was obtained with halothane. This suggests that in the presence of ventilation perfusion abnormality, the less soluble agent, nitrous oxide, desflurane, and sevoflurane may be delayed more than halothane or isoflurane.

Effect of N₂O in closed spaces

During anaesthesia appreciable volumes of N_2O can move into closed gas spaces without influencing F_A/F_I with important consequences. The closed gas spaces are enclosed by compliant or non-compliant walls; former subject to changes in volume secondary to the transfer of N_2O into these spaces[18] (bowel gas, pneumothorax or pneumoperito-nium). These spaces already contain N_2 (from air) with a low solubility (blood gas partition coefficient 0.015) which limits its removal by blood. The entry of N_2O is more than N_2 (air) removed, resulting in an increased volume. Theoretically, this volume expansion is a function of alveolar N_2O concentration. An alveolar concentration of 50% might double the gas space volume, and a 75% might produce a four-fold increase with a rapid increase. Administration of 75% N_2O in the presence of pneumothorax may double the pneumothorax by 10 minutes. And triple it by 30 minutes (Fig. 8)[19].

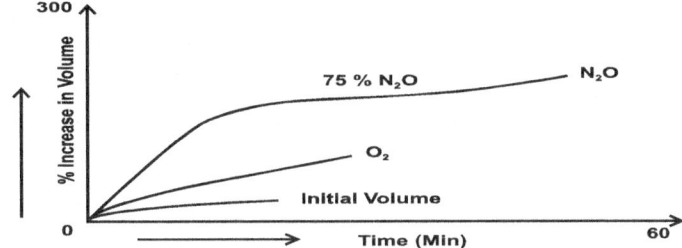

Fig 8: Initial volume of Pneumothorax, no effect of O_2, effect of 75% N_2O

This increase in volume may seriously impair cardiorespiratory function, and the use of N_2O is contraindicated in the presence of pneumothorax. If air inadvertently enters the blood stream, then there is still more rapid expansion of pneumothorax, especially when patient is breathing N_2O instead of air. This air embolus expands and is fatal. Air filled cysts of endotracheal tube can be increased three times in a short time.

N₂O in Poorly Compliant Spaces

The pressure may increase in such cavities, e.g., unwanted increase in intraocular pressure by N_2O administration after intravitreal sulphur hexaflouride injection. Other examples include the gas space created by pneumoencephalography and the natural space in the middle ear leading to ear pain[20]. The N_2O used in decreased tympanoplasty because increased pressure may displace the graft, or affect hearing.

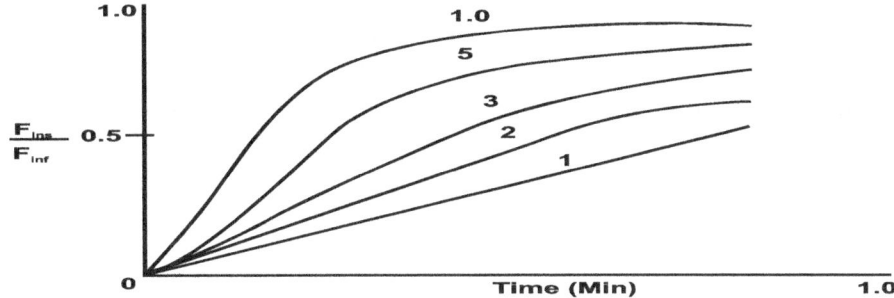

Fig. 9: Rate of increase in F_{ins} is determined by inflow rate and circuit volume

Anaesthesia Circuits

The rebreathing that results from the use of an anaesthetic causes inspired concentration to be less than that in the gas delivered from the machine. The rebreathing inspired concentration is influenced by the delivered concentration, by need to 'washin'in circuit and by depletion of anaesthetic in rebreathed gas after its uptake in lungs.

Washin Circuit

The anaesthetic may be washed into circuit volume i.e., corrugated hoses and rubber bags etc. at inflow rate of 1-5 litre/min and a circuit volume of 7 litres (bag 3 litres, CO_2 absorber 2 litres and corrugated tubes and fittings 2 litres) the washin of 75 – 100 % is complete in 10 minutes. High inflow rates produce a more rapid rise in inspired concentration (Fig. 9).[21]

Anaesthetic Loss to Plastic, Rubber and Soda Lime

The rubber or plastic component of the circuit may remove agent like methoxyflurane with high solubility in rubber (Table 2)[22], while halothane and isoflurane have little solubility. The normal moist (13–15% H_2O) CO_2 absorbent can slightly increase sevoflurane requirement by degrading each of these anaesthetics, by removing hydrogen fluoride, N_2O, desflurane and isoflurane are not materially degraded. Sevoflurane and halothane degradation produces toxic unsaturated compounds (compound A from sevoflurane is nephrotoxic)[23] Desicated absorbents degrade all anaesthetics.

Table 3: Rubber gas partition coefficient

Anaesthetic	Rubber bag	Polyvinyl	Polyethylene chloride
N_2O	1.2	—	—
Desflurane	19	35	16
Sevoflurane	29	68	31
Isoflurane	49	114	58
Enflurane	79	—	—
Halothane	190	233	128
Methoxyflurane	742	—	118

In addition dehydration of baralyme increases compound A in case of sevoflurane, while dehydration of soda lime does the opposite. Degradation by soda lime is minimal at hydrations, $1/10^{th}$ of those found in soda-lime.

Effect of Rebreathing

The patient taking up anaesthetic from rebreathed gas, the amount taken and the amount rebreathed, influences the anaesthetic concentration. Increased rebreathing lowers the inspired concentration of poorly soluble gas. This effect can be reversed by decreasing rebreathing and by increasing the inflow rate of 5 L/min[24]. High inflow rates of 5 L/min or more has the advantage of increased predictability of the inspired concentration, but have the disadvantages of wastage of gases, increased OT atmosphere pollution, lead to higher volatile agent consumption, result in dry inspired gases and a great difficulty in estimating ventilation from excursions of reservoir bag.

Low flows (closed circuit)

Less than 3 L/min, low inflows have the advantages including lower cost, increased humidification, reduced heat loss, decreased atmosphere pollution, better capacity to assess ventilation. It has the disadvantages about achieved oxygen levels in the presence of N_2O, patients also contributing nitrogen from body stores which can decrease inspired O_2 concentration. There can be increased carbon monoxide concentration and rebreathing of toxic products from the breakdown of volatile anaesthetics. Carbon dioxide absorbents can degrade both halothane and sevoflurane to toxic compounds[24]. However, most important disadvantage is lack of control that low flows and especially closed circuits have.

Closed Circuit Anaesthesia

The closed circuit represents an extreme of anaesthetic administration, frequently accomplished because few systems completely eliminate leakage of gas from circuit. A leak of 200 mL/min is deliberately applied during sampling of gases for oxygen, CO_2 and anaesthetic analyzers.

Usually closed circuit requires a replacement of O_2, N_2O and volatile agents. Oxygen replacement remains constant unless metabolic changes due to sympathetic responses, body temporarily shivering. N_2O replacement follow a fairly predictable course as its concentration usually does not vary and its insolubility in fat makes it more prone to percutaneous loss which is a constant value.

There is an enormous difference between delivered (vaporizer dial) and alveolar concentration in closed circuit. The difference decreases with less soluble agents, but after the initial high uptake period is passed, the diluted concentration markedly exceeds the alveolar concentration that it sustains. The changes in uptake (e.g., secondary to increase cardiac output resulting from surgical stimulus) can cause considerable alterations in alveolar concentration unless the delivered concentration is altered. The alveolar concentration changes for two reasons: 1. Assuming a constant variation, the difference between alveolar and inspired concentrations vary directly with uptake and 2. Because of the rebreathing the inspired concentration varies inversely with the uptake. Thus, the sum of these effects either decrease or increases the alveolar concentrations. A closed circuit has in inherent element of instability not present in an open circuit.

Low Flow Anaesthetic Delivery

The instability of closed circuit can be offset by use of low flow (less than half a minute ventilation) anaesthetic delivery. Low flow delivery has the advantage of economy, maintenance of humidification and temperature and limited O.T pollution. Low flow delivery also diminishes the disadvantages of the closed circuit in the constancy of oxygen and anaesthetic levels and toxic breakdown products. In low flow delivery system, concentration delivered from vaporizer (F_D) and that in alveoli (F_A) ratio governs the uptake. Thus F_D/F_A is higher for more soluble agents. This ratio is highest early in administration regardless of the solubility and decreases rapidly in the first 5 to 10 minutes of anaesthetic (as uptake by VRG tissues decreases to near equilibration), and more slowly thereafter (as uptake by muscles and fat decreases).

The inflow rate also governs F_D/F_A. The relationship is inverse. An increase in inflow rate decreases F_D/F_A by decreasing rebreathing (which decreases anaesthetic concentration in the rebreathed gases). Delivered gases concentration (F_D) must be sufficient to compensate for this depletion. The higher the inflow rate, the less the compensation required because of low rebreathing. But higher inflow rate do not produce proportional decreases in F_D/F_A. The greatest reduction in F_D/F_A comes with but modest increases in inflow rate. And once inflow rate exceeds minutes ventilation (a non rebreathing system exists) the further increase in inflow do not have effect on F_D/F_A which is same as the ratio of inspired (F_I) at alveolar concentration.

$$F_D/F_A = F_I/F_A.$$

High F_D/F_A provide a tight control over level of anaesthesia, produced by less soluble anaesthetic and higher inflow rates. The dial settings of vaporizer indicate the concentration of anaesthetic in the patient's lungs ($F_D = F_A$), but this is a poor correlation for all anaesthetics at all times, inflow rates etc. In fact delivered concentration is 20% greater than that in the alveoli (i.e., the F_D/F_A ratio is 1:2), even at inflow rates of 1–2L/min. If economy and low F_D/F_A ratio are desirable, the good compromise is to use a low flow delivery system after an initial period of higher inflow upto 1.5 minutes, at the time of highest uptake then decreased progressively as uptake decreases.

Table 4: Amount of liquid anaesthetic at various low flow rates.

Anaesthetic	Anaesthetic duration (min)	Inflow rate L/min 1.0	2.0	4.0
Halothane	30	4.5	5.4	8.0
	60	6.5	9.0	13.9	18.8
Isoflurane	30	5.8	8.0	12.3
	60	9.6	13.9	22.3	30.7
Sevoflurane	30	6.3	10.1	17.6
	60	10.9	18.2	33.0	47.8
Desflurane	30	14.8	25.0	45.2
	60	26.1	46.0	85.8	126

If the average inflow rate were 2L/min, 1 hour of anaesthesia with four potent anaesthetics listedin (Table 4)[25] would require administration of 9.0 to 40 mL liquid. This five fold range of values is smaller than eight fold range of potency.(MAC), since it must compensate for uptake and losses through overflow valve as well. The relatively smaller uptake and losses of the less soluble desflurane and isoflurane are what account for the reduction from eight fold to five fold. An even smaller range is focused at lower inflow rates, decreasing to about two fold for a closed circuit. However, such flows are not used with sevoflurane because of the greater concentration of compound A that results.

Recovery from Anaesthesia

All the factors governing the ratio at which alveolar anaesthetic concentration rises on induction apply to recovery. The immediate decline is very rapid. Only 2 minutes are required to eliminate 95–98% of N_2 from the lungs when 100% oxygen is given.

1. The rate of fall in alveolar concentration determines anesthetic recovery.
2. Increased solubility slows recovery
3. Increased cardiac output slows recovery
4. Increasing ventilation may help the recovery from potent agents, but with hyperventilation, the increased rate of fall in alveolar concentration is nearly balanced by the reduced cerebral blood flow.
5. Hyperventilation probably delays recovery from nitrous oxide, because there is little improvement in pulmonary wash-out, while wash-out from the brain is delayed from the reduced cerebral blood flow.

6. There is no concentration effect on emergence, as there was on induction, because the gas in high concentrations (nitrous oxide) is not being drawn from an infinite reservoir, as it was on induction.

Differences between induction and recovery

Recovery differs from induction where solubility hinders rise in alveolar concentration, could be overcome by increasing anaesthetic concentration. Such processes are seen during recovery, the inspired concentration cannot be reduced below zero. Secondly, on induction, all tissues have zero partial pressure of anaesthetic. During recovery the tissue partial pressures are variable. VRG pressures equals to that required for anaesthesia. The muscle group may or may not have same pressure as found in alveoli, specially with a shorter anaesthetic time. (1–2 hours). Fat group precludes equilibration of all the fat group with alveolar partial pressure with hours or even days, except in case in N_2O. Only when the alveolar (or arterial) anaesthetic pressure falls below that in tissue, it can contribute to anaesthetic to the alveoli. Thus recovery is rapid at first and expands upon the duration of anaesthesia [26].

Solubility influences the effect of duration of anaesthesia depending on the rate at which alveolar partial pressure declines.[26]

Diffusion Hypoxia

The uptake of large volumes of N_2O on induction of anaesthesia gives rise to concentration and second gas effects (Fig.10). On recovery, the outpouring of large volumes of N_2O can produce Fink phenomenon or diffusion anoxia.

These outpouring volumes cause displacement of oxygen and dilute alveolar CO_2 which decreases respiratory drive and hence ventilation. Because large volumes of N_2 are released only in first 5-10 minutes of recovery this period is of great concern as it is a time of maximum respiratory depression. To offset this 100% O_2 is administered in this period. This is more relevant in case of pre-existing lung disease or anticipated postoperative depression or after a narcotic, N_2O anaesthesia.

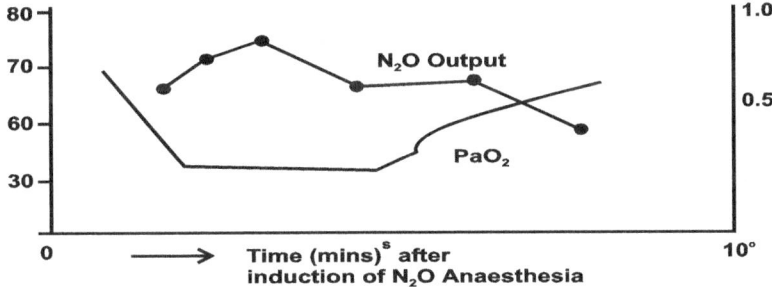

Fig. 10 : Effect of diffusion hypoxia on N2o output and PaO2

Impact of anaesthesia circuit

As in induction, the recovery can be affected by anaesthesia circuit. If patient is not disconnected from circuit on cessation of anaesthesia, the patient continues to inspire anaesthetic. For bringing down the inspired level to 0, several factors are accounted for. The anaesthetic within the circuit should be washed out, rubber or plastic components and soda lime within circuit will still have absorbed anaesthetic that will be released back into gas phase[21]. Which must be washed out. Finally anaesthetics coming out of exhaled air must be washed out. The effect of these factors to raise the anaesthetic concentration can be overcome by the use of high inflow rates of oxygen (greater than 5 litres).

Effect of metabolism

The saturation of enzymes responsible for metabolism may alter the rate of rise of alveolar partial pressure during induction but not during recovery. This metabolism may determine the rate at which alveolar partial pressure declines. The rapid ease with which halothane washout[12, 31] (15 – 20% recovered as urinary metabolites) as compared to enflurane(2–3 % recovered as metabolites during the course of anaesthesia). While halothane is eliminated through lungs and liver, enflurane via liver is minor. This also applies to desflurane, isoflurane and sevoflurane. Metabolism of first two is too small to accelerate their elimination, but the metabolism of sevoflurane is sufficient to narrow the difference between its washout and to that of desflurane[27].

Conclusion

1. In normal cases ventilation produces a rapid change (in and out of gases in the lungs).
2. When delivered concontration of anaesthetic is small (>10%), uptake opposes the effect of ventilation to quickly change the alveolar concentration of anaesthetic with F_I/F_A Inspired alveolar ratio is simple. If uptake remarks 80% anaesthetic the F_A/F_I is 0.2.
3. Uptake from lungs is a product of blood solubility, cardiac output and partial pressure of anaesthetic from lung to venous blood. Blood solubility determines F_A/F_I ratio and rate of induction and recovery from anaesthesia. Lower is the solubility, faster the recovery.
4. Anaesthetic depots formed by vesselrich group (VRG), muscle group (MG) and fat group (F.G.) They equilibration is faster in VRG (8 min) and slowest in FG. The difference in perfusion and equilibration determine the shape of F_A/F_I ratio.
5. Inspired inhaled anaesthetic concentration determines the F_A/F_I ratio (concentration effect). The later results from contracting of residual gases and an increase in inspired ventilation. These factors affect other gases given concurrently (second gas effect).
6. F_A/F_I is influenced further by metabolism and intertissue diffusion of anaesthetic. Other variables like ventilation, circulation, distribution of circulation, ventilation-perfusion abnormalities.
7. Low fresh gas flows provide economy, decreased pollution, heat conservation and humidification while a potential danger of rebreathing of toxic of different solubility and affect the required delivered concentration
8. Nitrous oxide increases the volume or pressure with gas containing spaces in the body.

REFERENCES

1. Steven L. Shafer, M.D: Inhalational Anesthetics: Uptake and Distribution , July 24, 2007.
2. Johnson JE. Uptake and distribution of inhalational anaesthetics. www.isakanyakumari.com/CASCO2012/CME/I A 2.
3. Anesthesia and Anesthesiology Teaching Site: http://www.anesthesia2000.com
4. Eger EI II. Uptake of inhaled gases. The alveolar to inspired anaesthetic difference. In Eger EI Editor. Anaesthetic uptake and action 2nd edition Baltimore, Williams and Wilkins, 1974; 77–94.
5. Yasuda N, Lockhart SH, Eger EI II et al. Comparison of kinetics of sevoflurane and isoflurane in humans. Anesth. Analg. 1991;72: 316–324.
6. Korman B, Mapleson WW. Concentration and second gas effects. Can the accepted explanation be improved? Br. J. Anaesth. 1997; 78:618–625.
7. Eger EI II, Smith RA, Robbins DD. The concentration effect can be mimicked by a decrease in blood solubility. Anesthesiology. 1978; 49:282–284.

8. Fossulaki A, Lockhart S, Freyer BA et al. percutaneous loss of desflurane, isoflurane and halothane in humans. Anesthesiology. 1991; 79:479–486.
9. Laster MJ, Taharis, Eger EI II et al. Visceral losses of desflurane, isoflurane and halothane in swine. Anesth. Analg. 1991; 73:209–212.
10. Carpenter RL, Eger EI II, Johnson BH et al. Does the duration of anaesthetic administration affect the pharmacokinetics of metabolism of inhaled anaesthetics in humans? Anesth. Analg. 1987; 66:1–8.
11. Yamamora H. The effect of ventilation and blood volume on uptake and elimination of inhalation anaesthetic agents in progress in anaesthesiology. Proceeding of 4th world congress of anaesthesiology, Amsterdam. Excerpta medica. International congress series 1968; 394–399.
12. Eger EI II, Balman SH, Manson ES. Effects of the age on the rate of increase of alveolar anaesthetic concentration. Anesthesiology. 1971; 35:365–372.
13. Belnitre E, Raco H. the pulmonary exchange of nitrous oxide and halothane in children. Anesthesiology. 1969; 30:388–394.
14. Eger EI II, Severinghaus JW. Effects of uneven pulmonary distribution of blood and gas on induction with inhalation anaesthetics. Anesthesiology 1964; 25:620–626.
15. Eger EI II, Saidman LJ. Hazards of nitrous oxide anaesthesia in bowel obstruction and pneumothorax. Anesthesiology. 1965; 21:61–66.
16. Stoelting RK, Lognecker DE. Effect of right to left shunt on rate of increase in arterial anaesthetic concentration. Anesthesiology. 1972; 36:352–356.
17. Saidman LJ, Eger EI II. Change in cerebrospinal fluid pressure during pneumoencephalography under nitrous oxide anaesthesia. Anesthesiology. 1965; 26:67.
18. Eger EI II. Effect of anaesthetic circuit on alveolar rate of rise in anaesthetic uptake and action. Baltimore; Williams Wilkins. 1974, 192–205.
19. Eger EI II, Larson CP Jr., severinghaus JW. The solubility of halothane in rubber soda lime and various plastics. Anesthesiology. 1962; 23; 356–359.
20. Eger EI II, Koblin DD, Bawlan T et al. Nephrotoxicity of sevoflurane versus desflurane in anaesthesia in volunteers. Anesth. Analg. 1997; 84:160–168.
21. Harper M, Eger EI II. A comparison of the efficiency of three anaesthesia circle systems. Andy 1976; 55:724–729.
22. Weiskopf RB, Eger EI II, Comparing the cost of inhaled anaesthetics. Anesthesiology. 1993; 79:1413–1418.
23. Stoelting RK, Eger EI II. The effects of ventilation and anaesthetic solubility on recovery from anaesthesia. An in vivo and analog analysis before and after equilibration. Anesthesiology. 1969; 30:290–296.
24. Eger EI II, Johnson BH. Rate of awakening from anaesthesia with I 653, halothane, isoflurane and sevoflurane. A test of the effects of anaesthetic concentration and duration in rats. Anesth. Analg. 1987; 66:977–982.
25. Mapleson WW. Quantitative prediction of anaesthetic concentrations in; uptake and distributions of anaesthetic agents. Paperium Kitz RJ (Eds) New York. McGraw Hill 1963; 109–119.
26. Newman MA, Weiskopf RB, Gong DH et al. Changing from isoflurane to desflurane towards the end of anaesthesia does not accelerate recovery in humans. Anesthesiology. 1998; 88;914–921.
27. Raco H, Salanitre E, Frumin MH. Dilution of alveolar gases during nitrous oxide excretion in man. J. Appl. Physiol. 1961; 16:723–728.

Chapter 3   DORSAL HORN RECEPTORS

Many neurotransmitters and neuro modulators were involved in the dorsal horn. Excitatory amino acid glutamate acts at N-methyl D-aspartate (NMDA) and non-NMDA receptors. e.g. AMPA (alpha amino3-hydroxy 5-methyl 4-isoxazdepropionic acid), kainate and metabotropic glutamate receptors[1] (Table).

Several peptides released by primary afferents e.g., substance P and neurokinin A (acting through neurokinin receptors) calcitonin gene related peptide, opioid receptors, GABA, serotonin and adenosine receptors are receptors involved in neurotransmission and neuro modulation.[2] These reduce or modify the nociceptive impulse and offer a multimodal choice for pain relief.

The opioids have been used for postoperative pain mainly, also used in malignant and non-malignant pain. Intrathecal or epidural drug delivery is dictated by operative procedure and projected duration of the need for analgesia. Epidural route is preferred following withdrawal of subarachnoid micro catheters following risk of post dural puncture, headache and CSF leakage. Opioid agonists possess different selectivity against different type of pain e.g., Mu against thermal pain, kappa against pressure or visceral pain(Butorphanol, buprenorphine)in case of the later drugs, response difference in sex occurs due to oestrogen-opioid interactions in the dorsal horn[3]. Morphine is used in the range of 1–6 mg and 0.1mg, fentanyl 0.025–0.1mg and 0.005–0.01mg by epidural and intrathecal route respectively. The respiratory depression remains a major side effect with the use of opioids.

Alpha 2 Agonists

Clonidine and adrenaline provide spinal analgesia in acute and chronic patients. It provides dose related anxiolysis, sedation and augments the quality and duration of peripheral nerve block with local anaesthetics. It is taken 2 mg epidurally and 150–450 microgram intrathecally. Side effects include hypotension and bradycardia which is not present with the more potent dexmeditodimine[4]. A dose of 0.35 mg/kg intrathecally provides motor blockade upto 177.2 minutes when used along with sensorcaine (Kumar et al). There was no haemodynamic or other side effects.

Cholinomimetics and Cholinesterase Inhi-bitors

Stimulation of cholinergic receptors is a mechanism of endogenous analgesia. The muscarinic agonists may have a role in producing analgesia e.g., cholinesterase inhibitor neostigmine. However, there is a poor effect to side effect ratio. Intrathecal (100 mg) produced nausea, vomiting and transient lower extremity weakness, which is dose related[5].

Benzodiazepines

Benzodiazepines enhance the effect of GABA upon $GABA_A$ receptors and produce analgesia, which is reversible with benzodiazepine antagonist flumazenil as well as the GABA antagonist bicuculline. Baclofen used for spasticity acts on $GABA_B$ while muscimal acts in $GABA^A$ receptors. In animal studies limited data on intrathecal and epidural midazolam suggests a potential neurotoxicity after a single dose [4].

Ion Channel Blockers

Because spinal nociception depends upon ion flux to trigger postsynaptic depolarization in dorsal horn neurons mu or delta opioid agonist inhibit potassium flux, kappa agonist inhibit calcium flux and local anaesthetics inhibit sodium flux. Calcium influx initiates the intracellular cascade of genetic and biochemical responses to pain. Calcium channel blockade potentiates opioid analgesia while suppressing opioid abstinence syndrome. L-type voltage calcium channel block (L- VSCC) may not provide effective analgesia when given alone but nimodipine potentiates morphine analgesia. However, N–type VSCC abound on neurons and its synthetic analogue SNX– 11 is a potent analgesic for morphine resistant pain of neuropathic or malignant origin. Side effects are nausea, orthostatic hypotension, headache, constipation and confusion. Preclinical data on potassium channel block also points towards analgesic effects[6].

Table 1: Dorsal horn receptor and peptides

	Presynaptic	Postsynaptic	Role	Drugs acting
Peptides	Glutamate Substance P	AMPA receptor (Na^+ influx) neurokinin-1 (IP3,DAG) NMDA(Mg^+, Ca^+, Na^+ outflow)	Central sensitization Long– term memory (increased)	Ketamine MK-801
Receptor	Opioid (k,mu,sigma) GABA B, 5HT 3 Benzodiazepines adenosine	GABA B,GABA A 5HT 1B alpha 2 adenosine	Decrease nociceptive input Increase alpha 2 Seratonin	Opioids noradrenaline Clonidine

NMDA Agonists

Ketamine blocks the open calcium channels on NMDA receptor complex. It has been used along with local anaesthetics and opioids to prolong postoperative analgesia without any respiratory depression. However, epidural/spinal ketamine produces a shorter duration of analgesia with possibility of psychomimetic effects.

Other NMDA open channel blockers e.g., dextro–metorphan, phencyclidine and glycine binding drugs have been used in experimental stages. Amitriptylline is found to suppress NMDA induced hyperalgesic states intrathecally in animals. It also enhances analgesia by augmenting the effects of noradrenaline and serotonin [4] (Fig. 1).

NSAIDS and Nitric Oxide Synthase Inhibitors

These inhibit intracellular enzymes activated by calcium entry into the postsynaptic cell (nitric oxide synthetase and phospholipase). These in turn generate nitric oxide and arachidonic acid, the latter being a substrate for cyclooxygenase isoenzymes, COX –1 and COX– 2. Spinal injection of NOS inhibitor L-NAME blocks thermal hyperalgesia as well as NMDA induced hyperalgesia. Lysine salicylate intrathecally provides analgesia for refractory cancer pain. Acetaminophen intrathecally provides analgesia and reversal of hyperalgesia [7].

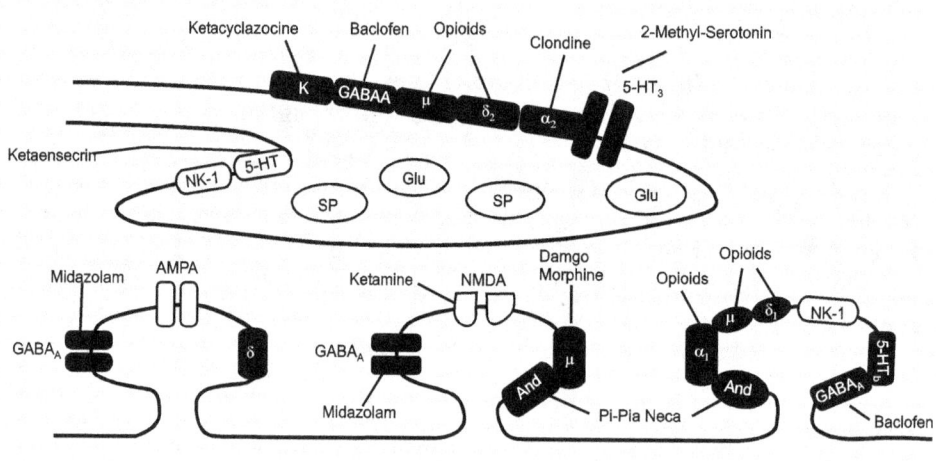

Fig1 : Dorsal horn receptors and drugs acting on it

Adenosine and Non Opioid Peptides

Adenosine receptors A1 and A2 are linked to analgesia, through spinal cord adenosine release, which if blocked by intrathecal theophylline producing hyperalgesia. Opioids and serotonin when used intrathecally release adenosine and produce analgesia.

Other peptides are substance P and related tachykinins like somatostatin, produce epidural/spinal analgesia[10,11]. However, histopathological changes in spinal cord may present which is dose related. A dose of 20 microgram may be neurotoxic in rats but doses below 15 microgram are not [9]. Its use was abandoned until its stable analogue octreotide produced analgesia in cancer patients by intrathecal infusion [4].

References

1. Wilcox GL. Excitatory neurotransmitter and pain. In bond MR, Charlton JE and Woolf CJ, Vol 4, pp 97–117, Amsterdam, Elsevier.
2. Bond MR, Charlton JE and Woolf CJ, (eds); Proceedings of 6th world congress on pain, Pain research and management series, Vol 4 pp 97– 117, Amsterdam, Elsevier, 1991.
3. Amandusson A, Hermansion O, Blomquist A, Estrogen receptor like immuno reaction in dorsal spinal horn and medulla of female rat. Neuroscience lett. 196; 25,1995.
4. Cousins MJ, and Bridenbaugh (Eds) Neural blockade in clinical anaesthesia and management of pain. 3rd edition, pp 946. Philadelphia, Lippincott Raven, 1998.
5. Kumar P, et el Clonidine with lignocaine or bupivacaine intrathecal in spinal analgesia. Ind. Journal of anaesthesia, 1993; 41:240–242.
6. Lauretti GR, Reis, Prado WA and Klampt JG. Dose response study of intrathecal morphine Vs intrathecal neostigmine, their combination or placebo for post op analgesia in patients undergoing anterior and posterior vaginoplasty. Anaesth Analg. 1996; 82–1182.
7. Malmberg AB, Yaksh TL. Antinociceptive actions of spinal NSAIDs on formalin test in rats. J. Pharm. Exp. Therapy, 1992; 163, 136.
8. Delander GE and Wahl JJ. Behaviour induced by putative nociceptive neurotransmitter is inhibited by adenosine or adenosine analogues co–administered intrathecally. J. Pharm. Exp. Therapy, 1988; 246–565
9. Chrubasik J, Meynadier J, Scherpereli P, et al. The effect of epidural somatostatin on post op analgesia, Anaesth,.Analg. 1985; 4:3085–3985.

Chapter 4. The Autonomic Nervous System

The ANS maintains the cardiovascular, gastrointestinal and thermal homeostasis. It provides involuntary control and organisation of both maintenance and stress response.

Activation of the sympathetic nervous system elicits the "fight or flight" responses, which includes redi-stribution of blood flow from the viscera to skeletal muscles, increased cardiac function, sweating, salivation and papillary dilatation.

The parasympathetic system governs activities associated with the maintenance of function, such as digestive and genitourinary functions.

Nerves are traditionally classified by the chemical transmitters they contain. Nerves containing acety-lcholine (Ach) are called cholinergic nerves, whereas those containing norepinephrine (noradrenaline in India) or epinephrine (adrenaline) are called adrenergic receptors and those receptors that react with Ach and cause the cell to respond in a characteristic way.

Cholinergic agonists are drugs that act like Ach on the cholinergic receptors. They are also referred to as cholinomimetic drugs. Cholinergic antagonists are drugs that react with the cholinoreceptors to block the acess by Ach and so prevent its action. These drugs are also known as cholinolytic cholinergic blocking or anti-cholinergic drugs. Muscarine a chemical isolated from a mushroom causes effects similar to those produced by activation of the parasympathetic nervous system. Drugs that mimic the effects of muscarine are called muscarinic drugs. Because muscarinic drugs act on the parasympathetic system, agonists are sometimes called parasympatho-mimetic drugs and antagonists are called parasympatho-lytic drugs.

Nicotine was found to act on ganglionic and skeletal muscle synapses, on nerve membranes and sensory endings. Drugs that act on these parts of the cholinergic system are called nicotinic drugs.

Cholinergic nerves include the following:
1. All motor nerves that innervate skeletal muscles.
2. All postganglionic parasympathetic neurons.
3. All preganglionic sympathatic and parasympathetic neurons.
4. Some postganglionic sysmpathetic neurons e.g., those innervating sweat glands and certain blood vessels.
5. Preganglionic sympathetic neurons that arise from the greater splanchnic nerve and innervate the adrenal medulla.
6. Central cholinergic neurons.

Drugs mimicking the action of noradrenaline (NA) are referred to as sympathomimetic, whereas drugs inhibiting these effects of NA are called sympatholytic. NA is the transmitter acting at adrenergic nerves, whereas both adrenaline and noradrenaline are released by the adrenal medulla. Adrenergic neurons include the following:
- Post-ganglionic sympathetic neurons.
- Some interneurons.
- Certain central neurons.

Apart from the classical transmitters i.e., NA and Ach other neurotransmitters have also been identified. They are: mono amines, purines, amino acids, polypeptides, ATP, vasoactive intistinal polypeptide (VIP) substance P(SP), 5-hydroxy tryptomine (5HT), neuropeptide Y (NPY) and calcitonin gene-related peptide (CGRP). The most common combination of transmitter in perivascular neurons are NA and NPY in sympathetic nerves; Ach and VIP in parasympathatic nerves and SP, CG RP and ATP in sensory motor nerve.

Sympathetic Nervous System

The sympathetic nervous system originates from the spinal cord in the thoracolumbar region, from the 1st thoracic through to the second or third lumbar segment. The preganglionic sympathetic neurons have cell bodies within the horns of the spinal grey matter. Nerve fibres from these cell bodies extend to three types of ganglia grouped as paired sympathetic chains, various unpaired distal plexus or terminal or collateral ganglia near the target organ.

The twenty two paired ganglia, lie along either side of the vertebral column. The pre ganglionic fibres leave the cord in the anterior nerve roots, join the spinal nerve trunks and enter the ganglion at that level via the white (myelinated) ramus. Leaving the ganglion post-sympathetic fibres enter the spinal nerve via the grey (unmyelinated) ramus, then either go on to innervate pilomotor and sudomotor (sweat gland) effectors blood vessels of the skeletal muscle and skin (Fig.1).

The sympathetic distribution to the head and neck comes from the three ganglia of the cervical sympathetic chain.

The unpaired prevertebral ganglia reside in the abdomen and pelvis anterior to the vertebral column and include celiac, superior mesenteric, aortico, renal and inferior mesenteric ganglia. Celiac ganglion, innervated by T_5 to T_{12} and innervates liver, spleen, kidneys, pancreas, small bowel and proximal colon. Superior mesenteric ganglion innervates distal colon.

Inferior Mesenteric Ganglion—innervates rectum, bladder and genitals.

Terminal or collateral ganglia are few and lie near the target organ.

Sympathetic preganglionic fibres are short, whereas postganglionic long. However, sympathetic nerves need not synapse solely in the ganglion of their origin, but can course up and down the paired ganglia of the spinal cord. Thus sympathetic response is not confined to segment from which the stimulus originates. Instead there is a diffuse discharge of the sympathetic system.

Parasympathetic Nervous System

The parasympathetic nervous system arises from cranial nerves III, VII, IX and X as well as from the sacral segments. The ganglia of the parasympathetic system occur proximal to or within the innervated organ. Thus the parasympathetic nervous system is more targeted and less robust.

Preganglionic fibres of the parasympathetic system originate from the mid brain, the medulla oblongata and the sacral part of the spinal cord.

Mid brain

Fibres arising from the mid brain synapse in the ciliary ganglion and innervate the smooth muscle of the iris and ciliary.

Medulla oblongata

Gives rise to parasympathetic components of the facial, glossopharyngeal and vagus nerves. Facial nerve supplies parasympathetic innervation to ganglion of the submaxillary and sublingual glands and sphenopalatine ganglion. The glosso pharyngeal nerve will ultimately innervate the mucous salivary and lacrimal glands. The vagus nerve supplies the heart, tracheobronchial tree, liver, spleen, kidney and all the gastrointesitnal tract except distal colon.

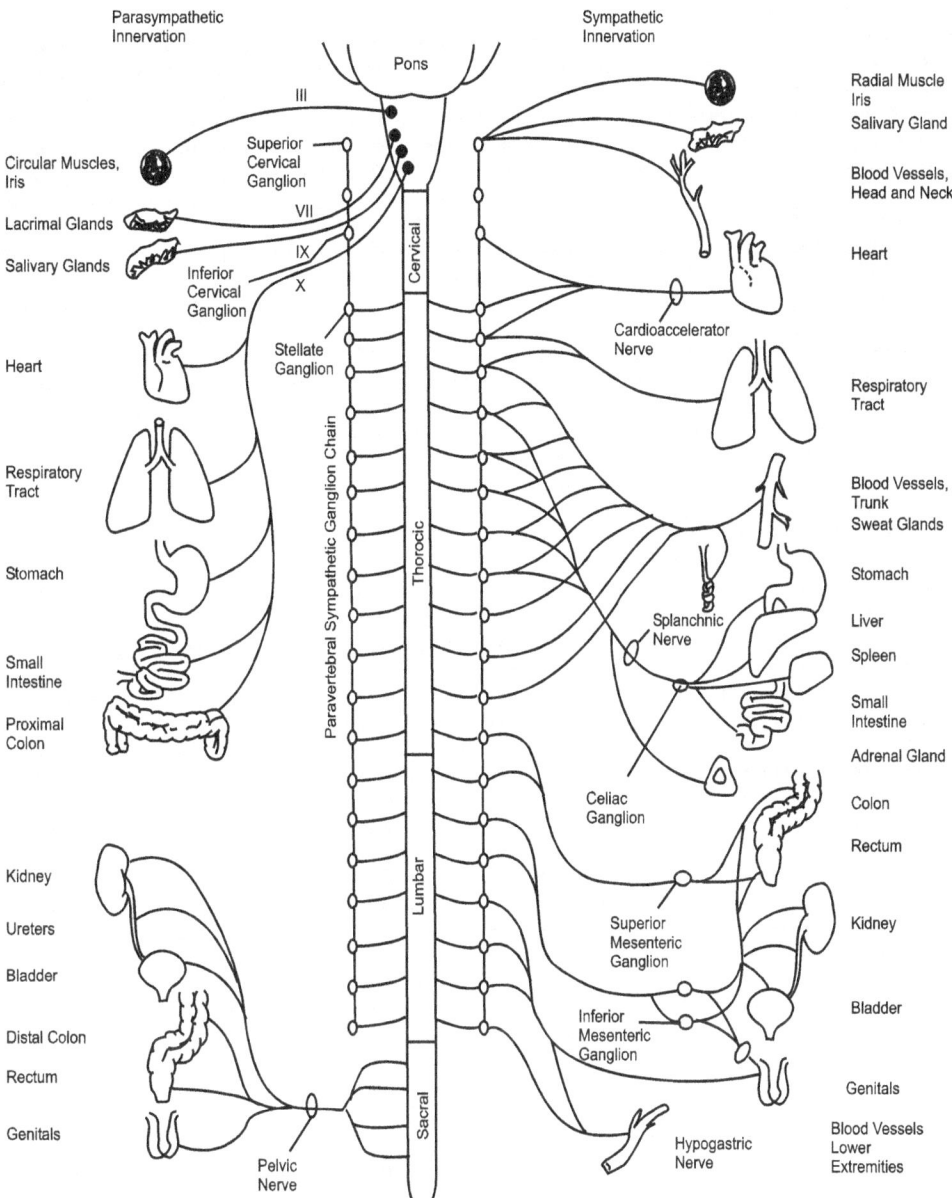

Fig. 1: Autonomic nervous system

Sacral segments

The 2nd through 4th sacral segment contribute the nervi erigentis, or pelvic splenic nerves. They synapse in terminal ganglia associated with the rectum and genito urinary organs.

Enteric Nervous System

The enteric nervous system is the system of neurons and their supporting cells found within the walls of the gastrointestinal tract including the neurons within the pancreas and gall bladder [3]. The enteric nervous system has an extra ordinary degree of local autonomy although it is still influenced by the sympathetic and parasympathetic activity. The sympathetic preganglionic fibres from T_5 to L_1 are inhibitory to gut action. Therefore spinal anaesthesia will yield a contracted small intestine with superior surgical conditions [4]. During abdominal surgery, when the viscera are handled, a reflex firing of the adrenergic inhibitory nerves inhibits the motor activity of the intestine. This can be the basis of postoperative ileus.

Certain plexuses that play a role in the enteric nervous system are myenteric plexus (Auerbach's plexus) and submucous plexus (Meissner plexus). These plexuses contain vesicles that are presumed to be store houses of neurotransmitters.

Acetylcholine is the principle excitatory trigger of the non sphincteric portion of the enteric nervous system, causing muscle contraction.

Function of ANS

The sympathetic system acts to increase the heart rate, blood pressure and cardiac output, to dilate the bronchial tree and to shunt the blood away from the intestine and other viscera to better the supply to the voluntary muscles.

The parasympathetic nervous system acts primarily to conserve energy and maintain organ function and to support the negative process.

Most organs exhibit a dual innervation frequently mediating opposing effects.

Adrenergic Function
Effects of Epinerphrine (Adrenaline)

Adrenergic neurons have been identified and subdivided into alpha-and beta-receptors and further subdivided into $alpha_{1-2}$-, $Beta_1$- and $beta_2$- receptors. $alpha_2$- receptors are primarily located on the parasympathetic membrane and $alpaha_1$-receptors mediate smooth muscle vasoconstriction. beta1 receptors are found primarily on cardiac tissue and beta2-mediate smooth muscle relaxation (Fig. 2).

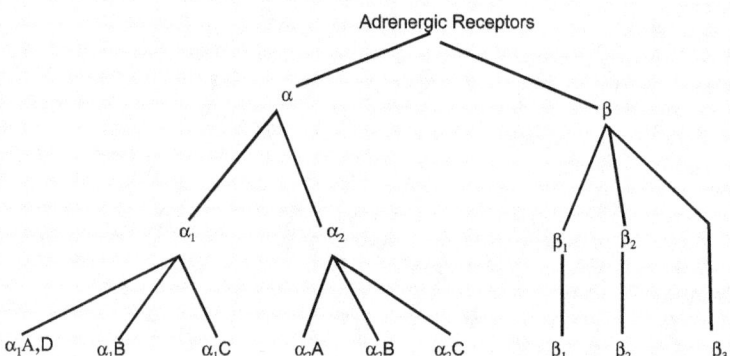

Fig. 2: Adrenergic receptors

Adrenergic neuron stimulation mainly affects the circulation and respiration. Ventilation is increased by central effect on ventilatory centres and bronchodilation. Cardiac output is increased through increased contractility of the heart and increased rate of contraction. Perfusion pressure for vital organs is increased function of gastrointestinal and genitourinary system is decreased.

Alpha receptor stimulation results in smooth muscle contraction including ciliary muscle and vascular smooth muscle [5]. The gastrointestinal and genitourinary sphincter is also stimulated.

Beta receptor stimulation results in stimulation of the heart, relaxation of vascular and bronchial smooth muscles and stimulation of renin secretion by the kidney. (Table.1)

Table 18. : Distribution of alpha-and beta-receptors

Receptors	Distribution	Response
alpha$_1$	Smooth muscle	Constriction
alpha$_2$	Presynaptic	Inhibit NE release
beta1	Heart	Inotropy and chronotropy
beta2	Smooth muscle	Dilation and relaxation

Cholinergic Function
Effects of Acetylcholine

The parasympathetic system is essential for the maintenance of life. All release is the hallmark of parasympathetic activation. Ach is the only endogenous compound that causes simultaneous bradycardia and hypotension.

The dose of Ach determines the effect or effects—a small IVdose causes generalized vasodilation, whereas a larger dose produces negative chronotropic and dromotropic effects. Ach decreases the rate of cardiac contraction. The velocity of conduction in SA and AV node and contractility in the atria. Cholinergic receptor stimulation of the endothelium releases EDRF (endothelium derived relaxing factors) causing vaso- dilation. But if the endothelium is damaged, cholinergic receptor stimulation causes vasoconstriction.

Ach stimulates the chemoreceptors. It also causes smooth muscle constriction including bronchial walls and iris causing miosis. In gastrointestinal and genitourinary tract there is constriction of smooth muscles in the walls but relaxation of the sphincters. Cholinergic overload can lead to nausea, vomiting, intestinal cramps, belching, urination and defecation.

Norepinephrine (Noradrenaline, NA)
Synthesis

Noradrenaline, NA is synthesized from tyrosine which is synthesised from phenylalanine. However, tyrosine is also available from the diet. A series of steps results in the conversion of tyrosine to NA and adrenaline.

The first step involves tyrosine hydroxylase (TH) which is the rate controlling step for NA biosynthesis. Tyrosine is converted by the enzyme TH to dehydroxyphenylalanine (DOPA) which in turn is decar-boxylated to dopamines by DOPA decarboxylase. Dopamine is b-hydroxylated within the vesicles to NA by the enzyme dopamine b-hydroxylase (DBH). In the adrenal medulla, phenylethanolamine N-methyl transferase (PNMT) methylates 85% of NA in adreneral medulla to adrenaline.

Storage

Noradrenaline, NA is stored within large, dense core vesicles. There appears to be an actively recycling population of sympathetic vesicles and a reserve population of vesicles that is mobilized only on extensive stimulation. Functionally NA is stored in compartments of which 10 per cent is readily releasable. On stimulation the contents of the vesicles are released into the sympathetic cleft. Approximately 10 per cent of stored epinephrine is resistent to depletion such as occurs with reserpine.

Release

There are two processes by which the contents of the vesicles enter the sympathic cleft. The first is by the leakage from the vesicles into the presynaptic cytoplasmic and subsequent release. This is known as the indirect release, occurring with ephedrine, bretylium, reserpine. The second mechanism is known as exocytosis in which the vesicles respond to the entry of calcium by initiating a process of vesicle docking, fusion and endocytosis [6]. Angiotensin II, prostacyclin and histamine may potentiate release, while Ach and prostaglandin E inhibit release. When an action potential reaches a nerve terminal the presynaptic plasma membrane depolarizes and the voltage gated calcium channels open at the active zone. Only small amount of calcium is required to initiate the process. The ensuing rise in intracellular calcium triggers exocytosis of synaptic vesicles resulting in the release of neurotransmitters [7]. The synaptic vesicle membranes are reclaimed from the plasma membrane by endocytosis and the vesicles eventually refill with neuro-transmitters. Exocytosis is distinct from the secretory process as it is a local pathway, independent of organelles and it occurs faster than secretions.

Inactivation

The Noradrenaline (NA) is removed from the synaptic cleft by (a) an amine uptake mechanism (uptake 1) (b) uptake by non neuronal tissue (uptake 2).

The majority of released NA is transported into the storage vesicles before. The neurotransmitter uptake into the synaptic vesicles is driven by, as electrochemical proton gradient across the synaptic membrane. Following reuptake, the small amounts of NE not taken up into the vesicles are deaminated by MAO. The reuptake mechanism is not specific for NA and other structurally similar compounds (false transmitters) may be taken up leading to depletion of NA. Highest rate of re-uptake is in the heart and lowest in the peripheral blood vessels. The lungs remove 25 per cent of NA that pass through their circulation. The re-uptake of NA is decreased at rest during sympathetic activation and with aging.

Metabolism

Noradrenaline, NA that escapes re-uptake is metabolised by MAO or catechol-O-methyl transferase (COMT). This metabolism occurs in the blood, liver and kidney [8]. Adrenaline is also metabolised by the same enzymes. The final end product is vanillyl mandelic acid (VMA). Because of its rapid clearance, the half-life of NA in the plasma is very short (<1 minute.)

Adrenergic Receptors

Adrenergic receptors are classified into three major subtypes and nine sub subtypes.

α_1 adrenergic receptors have been further sub-divided into α_1 AD, α_1 B and α_1 C - receptors. The α_2-receptors are further subdivided into α_2A, α_2B and α_2C - isoreceptors. The α_1-receptors are found mainly in the smooth muscle and α_2-receptors are expressed parasympathetically and even in non neuronal tissues. The α_2 receptors are found in peripheral nervous tissue, CNS, platelets, liver, pancreas, kidney and eye [10]. The relevance of sub classification is that these receptors are also selectively distributed *e.g.*, prostate gland contains mainly α_1A receptors. Therefore, selective α, A antagonist would be more beneficial for benign prostatic hypertrophy.

Receptors can be presynaptic as well as post synaptic. Presynaptic receptors may act as either hetero receptors or autoreceptors. An autoreceptor is a presynaptic receptor that reacts with the neuro-transmitter release from its own nerve terminal, providing feedback regulation of hetero receptors, is a presynaptic receptor that respond to substances other than the neurotransmitter release from that specific terminal.

β-Receptors

The β-receptor is one of the super family of proteins. β-receptors have been further classified into $β_1$, $β_2$ and $β_3$ subtypes, all of which increase cyclic adenosine monophosphate (cAMP) through adenyl cyclase and the mediation of G proteins [11]. Although traditionally $β_1$- receptors were isolated in cardiac tissue and $β_2$-to smooth muscle. It is now recognized that $β_2$-receptors in cardiac function is more important than indicated. $β_2$-receptors may play an important role in compensating for disease, helping to maintain response to catecholamine stimulation as $β_1$-receptors are down regulated [12]. In addition to positive inotropic effects, $β_2$- receptors in the human atria participate in the regulation of heart rate.

Dopamine Receptors

Dopamine acts as α, β and dopamine receptors. Dopamine receptors are divided into dopamine (DA_1) and dopamine 2α (DA_2) receptors. DA_1 receptors are post synaptic and act on renal, mesenteric, splenic and coronary vascular smooth muscle to mediate vasodilation. DA_2 receptors are presynaptic and their action may be to inhibit NA and perhaps Ach release. Central DA_2 receptors may mediate nausea and vomiting. The antiemetic effect of droperidol is related to its DA_2 activity.

G Proteins

After adrenergic receptors stimulation the extracellular signal is transformed into an intracellular signal transduction in which α–, and β– receptors are coupled to G proteins. When activated, the G proteins can modulate either the synthesis or the availability of intracellular second messengers. The activated second messenger differs through the cytoplasm and stimulate and enzymatic cascade.

Cholinergic Pharmacology
Acetylcholine Synthesis

Ach is synthesised intraneurally from acetyl coenzyme A (CoA) and choline via the enzyme choline acetyltransferase in the synaptosomal mitochondria. Source of choline include dietary phospholipids, hepatic synthesis of phosphatidylcholine and choline release by hydrolysis of Ach.

Storage and Release

The neuromuscular junction includes the nerve endings, the muscle and the synaptic cleft which is a space between the nerve and the muscle. On the nerve or presynaptic side, the nerve ending contains many synaptic vesicles (quanta) that contain Ach (Fig. 3).

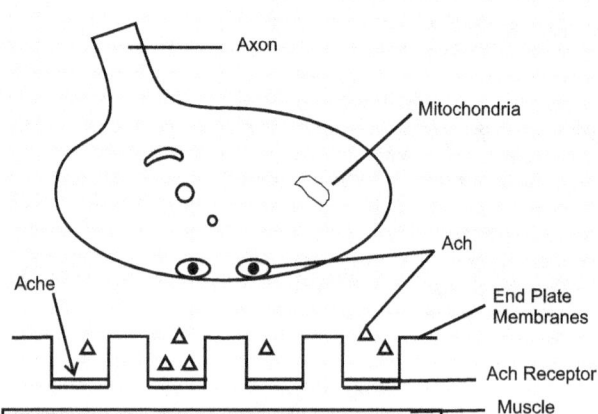

Fig. 3 : Parasympathetic division

On the muscle membrane there are many infoldings of the post junctional membrane. The presynaptic release sites are located opposite to the junctional folds. When a nerve impulse arrives at the presynaptic nerve terminal, it causes an influx of calcium ions across the membrane. This induces 100 to 300 synaptic vesicles to fuse with the presynaptic membrane, resulting in the liberation of Ach from vesicles into the synaptic cleft. The depolarization of the synaptic vesicles is known as endplate potential (EPP) or synaptic potential or excitatory postsynaptic potential (EPSP). The EPP (50 to 100 mV) triggers a muscle action potential. In the absence of a nerve impulse, there is a series of miniature endplate potentiates (MEP resulting from the spontaneous release of one quantum of Ach.

Inactivation

Ach is hydrolysed by acetylcholinesterase and butyrylcholin esterase. Acetylcholinesterase is a membrane bound enzyme that is present in all cholinergic synapses where it functions to destroy the neurotransmitter release from the nerve endings. Butyrylcholin esterase or pseudocholin esterase is made primarily in the liver and circulates in the blood. Its function in normal situations is not known. Butyrylcholinesterase is important for the destruction of some cholinergic drugs many of which are not destroyed by acetylcholinesterase.

Acetylcholine release, diffusion across the synaptic cleft, binding to receptors on endplate membrane and hydrolysis is by acetylcholinesterase (AchE) in the absence of blocking drug.

Inhibition of acetylcholinesterase prevents the distribution of Ach in cholinergic synapses so can activate all cholinergic systems simultaneously.

Cholinergic Receptors

Cholinergic receptors are divided into nicotinic and muscarinic receptors Muscarinic receptors are present in peripheral visceral organs, whereas nicotinic receptors are present on parasympathetic and sympathetic ganglia and neuromuscular junction of skeletal muscle. These two classes of receptors are structurally and functionally distinct and hence, this difference can be exploited by specific antagonists. Even the nicotinic receptors present on ganglia and motor endplate differ. The Ach receptors on the neuromuscular junction are receptor gated ion channels consisting of pentomeric membrane proteins. There are 2 α units and one each of β, ϵ and δ units. In order for the channel to open, Ach must occupy a receptor site on each of the α subunits. The ion channel response of Ach is instantaneous and usually lost only a few milliseconds. In adult skeletal muscle and postganglionic cells, choline receptors and their associated ion channels are present only in the immediate synaptic area and are absent from the rest of the cell membrane. When a nerve to a muscle is transacted it takes 1 to 3 days to increase the number of cholinergic receptors. These new receptors will no longer be confined to the motor endplate; this change has important clinical ramifications especially in burn induced denervation.

Muscarinic receptors are G protein coupled receptors. Muscarinic receptors utilize G proteins for signal transduction. Five muscarinic receptors utilize G proteins for signal transduction. Five muscarinic receptors exist (M_1 to M_5), selective muscarinic drugs, however, are not avoidable. Receptors in the muscarinic series are coupled to second messenger systems which in turn are coupled to ion channels. In other cases the influx of a cation is the trigger for a cellular response. In some cases an influx of calcium ions is initiated and these ions act as messengers that react with and open other ion channels *e.g.*, in cardiac atria activation of muscarinic receptors leads to the efflux of potassium and hyperpolarization of the cell membrane. In glands an influx of calcium and/or sodium activates intracellular events and causes the cells to secrete.

Drugs and the ANS

Pharmacologic manipulation of autonomic function is the basis of therapy in many acute and chronic illnesses and includes enhancement or inhibition of synthesis, storage or receptor mediated activity.

Drugs Affecting Adrenergic Transmission

Endogenous Catecholamines

Epinephrine (Adrenaline)

Adrenaline is used IV in life threatening circumstances like cardiac arrest, circulatory collapse and anaphylaxis. It can also be used locally to limit the spread of local anaesthetic or reduces blood flow.

Adrenaline activates all adrenergic receptors: $α_1$, $α_2$, $β_1$, $β_2$, and $β_3$. Effects of epinephrine includes positive inotropy, chronotropy and enhanced conduction in the heart ($β_1$), smooth muscle relaxation in the vasculature and bronchial tree ($β_2$), and vasoconstriction ($α_1$). Endocrine and metabolic effects of adrenaline include increased levels of glucose lactate and free fatty acids.

Bolus dose of 2 to 8 mg IV for pressure support. Bolus dose of 0.02mg/kg for cardiovascular collapse, asystole, ventricular fibrillation, anaphylactic shock and electromagnetic dissociation. For asystole and pulse less cardiac arrest in paediatric patients the initial dose is 0.01 mg/kg followed by 0.1 mg/kg every 3 to 5 minutes.

Endotracheal or intraosseous administration can also be done in the dose of triple IV dose and in diluted 10 mL, normal saline for endotracheal administration in adults [14].

For children 10 times the IV dose is required. Adrenaline should not be administered in alkaline solution because it gets rapidly degraded.

A rate of 1–2 µg/min predominantly activates $β_2$- receptors resulting vascular and bronchial smooth muscle relaxation. A rate of 2 to 10 µg (25 to 120 µg/kg/min) increases the heart rate, contractility and conduction through the AV node. Doses > 10 mg/min (100µg/kg/min) causes stimulation with generalised vaso-constriction.

Inhaled adrenaline was used in a 1% solution to treat bronchospasm. As it constricts oedematous mucosa, it is used in the treatment of severe croup and post extubation and traumatic airway oedema. A 2.22% solution is diluted with water or saline in 1:8 ratio and is nebulized.

Adrenaline is applied locally to mucosal surfaces to decrease bleeding in the operative field. It is mixed with local anaesthetics for infiltration. The α mediated vasoconstriction decreases bleeding and slows vascular update of local anaesthetic therapy prolonging its duration of action.

Relative contraindications include advanced age, significant tachycardia, hypertension and coronary occlusive disease.

Norepinephrine (Noradrenaline)

Noradrenaline (NA) acts at both α -and β -receptors but is usually used for its potent α agonism. It is the pressor of last resort in supporting the systemic vascular resistance. Less than 2 µg/min(30ng/kg/min) may uncover $β_1$ stimulation greater than 3 µg/min (50 ng/kg/min) elicit peripheral vasoconstriction from α stimulation and increases the blood pressure and may cause reflex bradycardia [15]. It also causes increased venous return; increased oxygen consumption unchanged or decreased cardiac output and may increase pulmonary vascular resistance.

Noradrenaline, NA is a potent constrictor of renal and mesenteric vascular beds and can cause renal failure, mesenteric infarction and peripheral hypo perfusion. The decreased hepatic blood flow can cause increased levels of hepatically metabolised drugs. Extravasation can cause tissue necrosis and may be treated with local infiltration of phentolamine, prolonged infusion can cause gangrene of the digits.

Dopamine

Dopamine acts at α, β and dopaminergic receptors. It also acts to release NA. Its main effect is to cause peripheral vasodilation. It is rapidly metabolised by MAO and COMT and has a half- life of one minute. It is, therefore, given as a continuous IV infusion. At doses of 0.5 to 2.0µg/kg/min, DA_1 receptors are stimulated and renal and mesenteric vascular beds are dilated [16]. At rates of 2 to 10 µg/kg/min, $β_1$- receptors are stimulated, leading to increased cardiac contractility and output. At 10 to 20µg/kg/min both α- and β- receptors are stimulated but the alpha vasoconstriction effect predominates. Dopamine is useful in the treatment of shock, CHF and cardiogenic shock.

Dopexamine is a synthetic dopamine analogue which is 60 times more potent at β_2-receptors, one third at DA_1, receptor with no and negligible β_1 effects. Fenoldopam is a selective DA_1 agonist and a potent vasodilator.

Non Catecholamine Sympathomimetic Amines

Most non catecholamine sympathomimetic amines act at α– and β– receptors and have two mechanisms of action: directly on a receptor and indirectly by releasing endogenous noradrenaline.

α Agonists

Phenylephrine and methoxamine are selective α_1 agonists and are used when peripheral vasoconstriction is needed, as a mydriatic and nasal decongestant. Clonidine is an example of an α_2 agonist. The primary effect is sympathetic lytic and they reduce peripheral noradrenaline release. These drugs are used as antihypertensive drugs. These drugs have also been used to attenuate the rise in intraocular pressure associated with laryngoscopy and endotracheal intubation. The α_2 agonists also provide effective analgesia for acute and chronic pain. Clonidine has also been used as an antiemetic and to treat panic disorders.

β Agonists

Non Selective b blockers include dobutamine and isoproterenol.

Although dobutamine acts on both α_1 and β_2 receptors it predominantly has β_1 effects. Dobutamine is useful in CHF and MI. It increases the cardiac contractility while lowering the filling pressures and does not increase the size of the infarct or cause arrhythmia [17]. Tachycardia is its primary side effect. Prolong treatment causes down- regulation of β-receptors and tolerance to its haemodynamic effect it is significant after 3 days.

Isoproterenol is a pure non selective β agonist. It is used to treat bronchospasm and it can cause tachycardia and arrhythmia as a side effect.

Selective β2 Agonists

These drugs are used primarily to treat bronchospasm. However, selectivity in dose dependent and is lost at higher doses. β_2 agonists are also used to treat premature labour. However, these drugs can cause tachycardia, increase susceptibility to arrhythmias and increased airway hyper reactivity *e.g.*, metaproterenol, albuterol and terbutaline.

α- receptor Antagonists

These drugs are utilized clinically as antihypertensive. They block the effect of endogenous catecholamines on arterial and venous constriction, reflex tachycardia and fluid retention.

Phenoxy benzamine is a prototype α₁-antogonist. Effects include decrease in peripheral resistance, increases cardiac output, blood flow to skin and viscera is increased. Side effects include orthostatic hypotension and nasal stiffness. Other α–receptor antagonists include phentolamine and prazocin and yohimbine.

β- receptor Antagonists

Indication for use of β blocker include IHD, post infarction management, arrhythmias, hypertrophic cardiomyopathy, hypertension and prophylaxis of migraine, headache. Competitive inhibition at the β– receptors can be overcome by increasing the available concentration of β agonists.

Nonselective beta blockers act at both β₁- and β₂- receptor: These include proprenolol, nadolol, pindolol, sotalol etc. Cardio selective beta blockers have a stronger affinity for β₁ than β₂-receptors. Cardio selective agents include atenolol, betaxolol, esmolol, metaprolol and becantolol. These drugs are preferred in patients with obstructive pulmonary disease, peripheral vascular disease, Reynaud phenomenon and diabetes mellitus. Labetolol vasodilates by blocking α₁- receptors as well as by direct β₂ agonism.

Some β blockers exert a partial agonist effect at the receptor while blocking access by more potent agonists and hence possess intrinsic sympathomimetic activity. These include acebutalol, pindolol, penbutolol etc. These agents lower the blood pressure with less decrease in resting heart rate and left ventricular function. Useful in patients with bradycardia.

Lipid solubility also affects absorption and metabolism. Propranolol metaprolol and pindolol are the most lipid soluble agents and hence their IV dose is much lower than their oral dose.

Adverse effects include bradycardia, asystole, decreased contractility, bronchospasm. Diabetes mellitus is a relative, contraindication because these drugs can mask the hypoglycaemia.

Drugs that inhibit synthesis, storage or release of noradrenaline: α Methyldopa acts by replacing NA in the nerve ending with a much less potent false neurotransmitter.

Reserpine: Affects the uptake of NA at the vesicular membrane, thereby inhibiting transport and storage of NA and dopamine, guanethidine and bretylfium. It is taken up into the adrenergic nerve ending and depletes NA stores after initially blocking release of NA.

Reserpine : Affects the uptake of NA at the vesicular membrane, thereby inhibiting transport and storage of NA and dopamine, guanethidine and bretylfium. It is taken up into the adrenergic nerve ending and depletes NA stores after initially blocking release of NA.

MAO and COMT: These enzymes are important in the degradation of catecholamines. MAOI binds irreversibly to the enzyme and causes increased amine concentration. This increase is associated with antihypertensive, antidepressant and antinarcoleptic effects.

Cholinergic Drugs: Drugs that affect para-sympathetic system act in one of the four ways.

1. Agonist stimulating cholinergic receptors.
2. Antagonist blocking or inhibiting the actions mediated by the cholinergic receptors.
3. Blocking or stimulating receptors on autonomic ganglia.
4. Inhibiting the metabolism of Ach thus increasing and prolonging the effect of Ach.

Agonists

Cholinergic agonists in clinical use have been derived from Ach, but they resist hydrolysis by cholinesterase, permitting a useful duration of action. Methacholine and bethanechol are primarily muscarinic agonists; carbachol has both nicotonic and muscarinic effects. Methacholine is used for diagnosing hyperreactive airways. Bethonechol is used postoperatively to reinstitute peristaltic activity in the gut or to force the extrusion of urine from an atonic bladder. Carbochol is used topically or intraoccularly to constrict the pupil for the long- term treatment of wide angle glaucoma.

Muscarine Antagonists

Muscarine antagonists compete with neurally released Ach for access to muscarine cholinoceptors and block its effects. They are also antagonists to the actions of muscarine agonists. The addition of a muscarinic anticholinergic drug to anaesthetic premedication to decrease secretions and to prevent harmful vagal reflexes, was mandatory in the era of other anaesthetics but is no longer necessary with modern inhalational agents. e.g., Atropine is a tertiary structure that easily crosses the blood brain barrier. CNS effects have been seen with relatively large doses. In contrast glyco-pyrrolate and synthetic antimuscarinic, does not cross the blood brain barrier and has a longer duration of action. Scopolamine is similar to the other drugs but has pronounced CNS effects. Ipratropium a muscarinic antagonist is useful in asthma and bronchospastic disorders [18]. The toxic effect of muscarinic antagonists is due to the blockade of muscarinic receptors in the periphery and in the CNS.

CNS effects include hallucinations, delusions, delirium and severe psychosis. These effects are reversible.

Atropine and scopolamine toxicity have been treated by physostigmine. Physostigmine must be administered with care because of its potentially lethal nicotinic effects which are not prevented by muscarinic antagonists.

Cholinesterase Inhibitors

Anticholinesterase drugs are used to produce sustained systemic cholinergic agonism. These drugs are used to reverse neuromuscular blockade, to treat myasthenia gravis and certain tachyrhythmias. First anticholine-sterase available was physostigmine. There are three classes of compounds used as cholinesterase inhibitors: carbonates, organophosphates and quaternary ammonium alcohols.

Physostigmine, neostigmine and pyridostigmine are carbamates and edrophonium is a quaternary ammo-nium alcohol. Organophosphate includes diso-propylfluorophospate, parathion ,malathion, somano-serin and a variety of other compounds used as insecticides.

Ganglionic Drugs
Agonists

These drugs are essential for analyzing the mechanism of ganglionic function but they have no therapeutic use.

Antagonists

These drugs were used to treat hypertension but because of interference with transmission through both the sympathetic and parasympathetic ganglia, anti-hypertensive action was accompanied by numerous side effects. Drugs in this class include hexamethonium, trimethaphan. Trimethaphan has a quick onset and short duration of action and hence it is useful for moment to moment control of blood pressure, hypertensive encephalopathy and controlled hypotension.

Clinical Syndromes-*Diabetes Mellitus*

It is the most common cause of autonomic neuropathy: Early small fibre damage is revealed by loss or impairment of vagally controlled normal heart rate variability, decreased peripheral sympathetic tone with subsequent increase in blood flow and diminished sweating, can also lead to diabetic neuropathic foot. Mechanisms maintaining normal standing blood pressure are altered.

Autonomic changes with aging

Aging is associated with alterations in vascular reactivity manifest clinically as exaggerated changes in blood pressure namely hypertension and orthostatic hypotension. Heart rate responses to changes in blood pressure, Valsalva manoeuvre and the respiratory cycle are blunted with aging[19].

Autonomic Changes in Spinal Cord Transection

Spinal cord transection may not only effect motor and sensory functions, but may also exhibit, profound alterations in autonomic activity that can alter anaesthetic care.

In cervical spinal cord transection, sympathetic and parasympathetic outflows are detached from central control mechanisms and this results in profound abnormalities altering the cardiovascular, thermo- regulatory, gastrointestinal and urinary systems.

In patients with high thoracic lesions, supine blood pressure is usually low with low plasma catecholamine levels. Patients with low spinal injuries exhibit compensatory tachycardia.

In patients with high spinal transection, tracheal suctioning can lead to unopposed vagal stimulation contributing to profound bradycardia. The phenomenon of autonomic dysreflexia can occur when stimulation occurs below the lesion, such as bowel or bladder distension. This autonomic reflex includes a dramatic rise in blood pressure, a marked reduction in flow to the periphery and flushing and sweating in areas above the lesion.

Thermogenesis is also impaired in spinal cord transection and hypothermia or hyperthermia can occur.

Summary

The ANS works in concert with renin, cortisone, and other hormones to respond to internal and external stresses.

The hallmark of the sympathetic system is amplification; the landmark of the parasympathetic nervous system is targeted responses.

Inhaled and intravenous anaesthetics can after haemodynamics by influencing autonomic function.

β-adrenergic blockade has emerged as an important prophylaxis for ischaemia and as a therapy for hypertension, MI and CHF.

The sympathetic nervous system demonstrates as acute and chronic adaptation to stress presynaptically and postsynaptically (*e.g.*, biosynthesis, receptor regulation).

Prestraptic α-receptor play an important role in regulating sympathetic release.

Many therapies for the treatment of hypertension are based on direct or indirect effects of sympathetic functions.

The vagus nerve is the superhighway of para-sympathetic function, accommodating 75% of para-sympathetic traffic.

Aging and many disease states (*e.g.*, diabetese, spinal cord injury) are accompanied by important changes in autonomic functions.

REFERENCES

1. Burstock G. The first von Euler lecture in physiology: The changing face of autonomic neurotransmission. Acta Physiol Scand 1986;126:67;1986.
2. Burns Tock G. Autonomic neuromuscular junctions: Current developments and future directions. J Anat 1986;46:1.
3. Lundberg JM. Evidence for coexistence of vasoactive intestinal polypeptide (VIP) and acetylcholine in neurons of cat exocrine glands: Morphological, biochemical and functional studies. Acta Physical Scand Sppl 1981;112:1.
4. Brindo baugh PO, Greene NM. Spinal (subarachnoid) neural blockade. In: Counsins M, Bridenbaugh P (eds): Neural Blockade in Clinical Anaesthesia and Pain Management. 2nd ed. Philadelphia JB Lippincott, 1988;213.
5. Lefkowithz R, Hoffman B, Taylor P. Drugs acting at synaptic and neuro effectors junctional sites. In Gilman A, Roll T, Nies A, et al (eds): Goodman Gilman. The pharmacological basis of Therpapeutics 9th En, New York, McGraw-Hill co 1996.
6. Shepherd J Von Houtte P. Neurohumoral regulation. In Shepherd S, Vanhoutte P (eds). The human cardiovascular system: Facts and concepts. New York, Raven Press, 1979; 107.
7. Katz B. Nerve muscle and synapse. Newyork, McGraw Hill 1966.
8. Lake CR, Chernow B, Feuerstein G, et al. The sympathetic neurons system in man, its evaluation and the measurement of plasma norepinephrine. In Ziegler M, Lake C (eds): Frontier of clinical neuro science Ballimore, Williams and Wilkins 1984;2:1.
9. Lauo Head R, Laall H, Bylund. D_2A Is the predominant a_2 adrenergic receptors subtype in human spinal cord. Anaesthesia 1993;77:983.
10. Szabo B, Hedler L, Stroke K. Peripheral presynaptic and central effects of cholindine, Yohimbine and rauwolcine, in the sympathetic nervous system in rabbits. Naunyn Schmiedeberg Arch Pharmacol 1989;340:648.
11. Raymond J, Hratowich M, Lefkowitz R, et al. Adrenergic receptors: Models for regulation of signal transduction processes. Hypertension 1990;15:119.
12. Opid LH. Ventricular overload and heart failure: In Opid LH (ed): The heart: Physiology and metabolism 2nd ed. Newyork Raven Press 1991;386.
13. Insel PA. Adrenergic receptors: Evolving concepts and clinical implications. N Engl J Med 1996;334:580.
14. Aitken had A. Drug administration during CPR: What route, Resuscitation 1991;22:191.
15. Zaritsky A, Chernow B. Catecholamines, sympathetomimetics. In Chernow B, Lake C (eds). The pharmacologic approach to the critically ill patient Baltimore, Williams and WIlkins 1983;481.
16. Goldberg L. Dopamine: Clinical uses of an endogenous catecholamine. N Engl J Med 1974;291;707.
17. Gillespie T, Amboo H, Sohel B et al. Effects of dolsestamine in patients with acute myocardial infarction. Am J Cardiol 1977;39:588.
18. Gross JN. Ipratropium bromide: N Engl J Med 1988;319;486.
19. Dares HEF. Respiratory changes in heart rate, sinus arrhythmia in the elderly. Gerontol Clin 1975;17:96.
20. Kumar Pramod. Equipments, Drugs & waveforms in Anaesthesia. 1st Edn, New Delhi, CBS Publishers, 2007.

CHAPTER 5. Inhalational & Intravenous Anaesthetic Agents

The continued dominance of inhalation methods of anaesthesia over regional and intravenous technique is attributed to many factors but particularly to their inherent safety and almost universal acceptability. Because of this and the fact that new inhalational agents are in the process of development and introduction, it is proposed to state briefly the properties. we should anticipate of the ideal inhalational agent.

Ideal Inhalational Agent[1]

- Pleasant and rapid induction with rapid emergence.
- Should be non-inflammable and chemically stable during storage and while in contact with all materials used in construction of anaesthetic circuits.
- Should be biochemically stable and non-toxic to parenchymatous organs even with prolonged use.
- It should be capable of inducing unconsciousness or sufficiently deep hypnosis to ensure amnesia.
- It should be sufficiently potent as an analgesic to prevent pain perception due to surgical stimuli.
- It should produce some degree of skeletal muscle relaxation.
- It should have high oil solubility and low water solubility.

Minimum Alveolar Concentration (MAC)

MAC is the minimum alveolar concentration of anaesthetic at 1 atmosphere that produce immobility in 50% of those patients exposed to a noxious stimulus [2]. The importance of MAC is as follows:

- MAC is the most readily measured index of partial pressure of drug at the anaesthetic site of action; the brain.
- MAC appears to be equally applicable to all inhalational agents and does not rely on fickle physical signs on side effects.
- MAC provides a useful number for the clinician in describing the dose of drug required to achieve the essential end point of anaesthesia; and analgesia.

Nitrous Oxide (N_2O)

Introduction

N_2O was first prepared by Priestly in 1772[3] but its anaesthetic properties were first demonstrated by Sir Humphry Davy in 1800.

Preparation

In the laboratory: Small amounts may be prepared by allowing iron to react with nitric acid. Nitric oxide i.e., NO is first produced, but this is reduced to nitrous oxide by an excess of iron.

$$2 NO + Fe \rightarrow FeO + N_2O$$

Commercially

Nitrous oxide is produced by heating ammonium nitrate to between 245°C to 270°C [4].

The process involved in making of the gas by British Oxygen Company in UK is as follows:

- A strong solution of ammonium nitrate when heated produces nitrous oxide with ammonia, nitric acid, nitrogen and traces of nitric oxide (NO) and nitrogen dioxide (NO_2).
- Cooling of the emerging gases results in reconstitution of ammonia and nitric acid to ammonium nitrate and this is returned to the reaction.

- Now gases are passed through water scrubbers which remove residual ammonia and nitric acid and then through potassium permanganate scrubbers which remove the higher oxides of nitrogen to leave a residuum of 1 VpM of nitric acid and nitrogen dioxide with purified nitrous oxide and some nitrogen.
- Acid scrubbers now remove any final traces of ammonia and gases are then compressed and dried in aluminium driers.
- About 9/10th of the contents of a full nitrous oxide cylinder are in liquid form. Great care is taken to prevent moisture being included in the cylinder contents, since water vapour tends to freeze as it passes through a reducing valve and may lead to obstruction of gas flow.
- When a nitrous oxide cylinder is turned on the gas tension within is first reduced and then rapidly increases again as some of the liquid vaporises.
- When flow rates of 10 L/min are used, there is a sharp linear fall in pressure, whereas only a small but nevertheless progressive fall occurs with a flow rate of 2 L/min.
- Pressure gauges on nitrous oxide cylinders would not indicate total contents until all the liquids is exhausted. They don't warn against failure of flow.
- Latent heat is required for the vaporization of the liquid nitrous oxide and it is obtained from the casing of the metal cylinder which as a result rapidly cools. This is turn leads to freezing of the water vapour in the air immediately surrounding the cylinder and thus forming a layer of ice on the cylinder.
- Nitrous oxide cylinders are available in various sizes and are coloured blue.

Physical Properties

- Non-irritating, sweet smelling and colourless.
- Only inorganic gas in regular use today.
- Molecular weight: 44.0.1
- Specific gravity: 1.527.
- Boiling point: –89°C
- Oil/water solubility ratio: 3.2
- Blood/gas solubility coefficient: 0.47
- Neither inflammable nor explosive.

Pharmacological Actions

Nitrous oxide will be rapidly absorbed in the alveoli and 100 mL of blood will carry 45 mL of nitrous oxide in its plasma.

1. Anaesthetic Action: Nitrous oxide is a weak anaesthetic having a MAC of 105. A 50:50 mixture of nitrous oxide and oxygen at 2 atm pressure rapidly produces surgical anaesthesia with complete oxygen saturation of the arterial blood, whereas the same concentration at atmospheric pressure in these patients did not produce loss of consciousness [5]. When nitrous oxide alone is used to induce anaesthesia, loss of consciousness is rapid enough—about 60 seconds, to suggest that this is primarily caused by displacement of oxygen from the blood rather than by saturation with nitrous oxide to a degree sufficient to cause anaesthesia without hypoxia. However, when accompanied with at least 33½% O_2 it has proved an immensely valuable supplement to other anaesthetic agents.
2. Circulatory effects: It has myocardial depressant properties and profound hypotension in patients who are anaesthetised with oxygen and halothane [6]. In clinical practice it would appear more reasonable to ignore the possibility that nitrous oxide may be associated with cardiovascular depression.

Metabolism and Toxicity

A. Hematological: Pancytopenia (aplastic anaemia) with a megaloblastic blood picture in patient given N_2O 50% for long period [7]. The severity of the megaloblastic marrow depression was directly related to the duration of N_2O inhalation: mild depression after 6 hours became severe after 24 hours. The mechanism is probably due to N_2O induced inactivation of vitamin B_{12} which leads to impaired methionine and deoxythymidine synthesis and defects in folate metabolism, all needed for normal haemopoisesis. The cobalt in the ring of B_{12} is catalytic in a reaction in which N_2O acts as a two electron oxidising agent.

Two Moles of B_{12} are oxidised by 1 mole N_2O.

B. Neurological: These have been reported in long term unintentional inhalation of N_2O as an environmental contaminant by dentists and his assistants. Signs are in the form of motor, sensory, coordination and reflex defects. This is also due to neuropathy caused by vitamin B_{12} lack. The failure to synthesize adenosyl methionine from methionine and ATP leads to failure of methylation of basic proteins in myelin sheaths, in particular, there is impaired methylation of arginine 10%.

C. Gestational: There is increased abortion rate among female assistants and among the wives of dentists. The main cause is through inactivation of B_{12} and in turn the effect on folate metabolism. When N_2O is given for periods more than 6 hours, neurological for periods more than 6 hours, neurological and haematological defects may occur.

Contraindications

There are no contraindications to the use of nitrous oxide in combination with an adequate % of oxygen. A minium concentration of 30% oxygen is recommended when nitrous oxide is used for anesthetic purposes.

Methods of Administrations

A. Intermittent flow: This is an economical method as gas flows only during inspiration, and it is based upon two different techniques.

(i) This technique depends on nitrous oxide and oxygen flowing into a mixing bag from which the patient inspires via corrugated tubing and mask. As the bag empties, it is refilled from the cylinder and when it is full, the flow of gases is automatically cut off until the next inspiratory effort starts the process once more. Mostly used in midwifery and dental practice.

(ii) Here a premixed cylinder of N_2O and O_2 under pressure with a demand valve to allow a high flow of gas to the patient on inspiration. The premixing of these gases in the same cylinder was suggested by Barach and Rovenstine and is reintroduced recently.

B. Continuous flow: A semi-closed system is used mostly with almost all expired gases passing into the atmosphere through the expiratory valve[7]. A completely closed system with absorption of CO_2 is not indicated when nitrous oxide is used, since it may be extremely difficult to ensure adequate oxygenation of the patient.

In the past inhalational agents like ethylcholoride, ether, trichloroethylene was in much use. The ethyl chloride spray was used as induction agent with open mask and later on maintenance was switched over to diethyl. The ethylchloride was highly cardiotoxic so its use was abandoned. Till lst 10 years ether was used in Boyel's anaesthesia machine through bottle ether vaporiser or through EMO vaporiser. The high incidence of nausea, vomiting, and secretions and introduction of more pleasant smelling halothane lead to the abandonment of the use of ether. The stages of ether anaesthesia were used as a typical teaching and chemical means for a typical anaesthesia technique. The availability of more accurate vaporiser also led to the use of halogenated inhalational agents. Ether was not suitable in varying temperatures and led to convulsions.

Diethyl Ether ($CH_3CH_2 - O - CH_2 - CH_3$)

Ether here is discussed for the sake of postgraduates and some of anaesthetists in remote area to give them theoretical knowledge and a sense of history and for examinations.

Manufacture

The concentrated sulphuric acid is mixed with 95 per cent alcohol and heated to 130° C. in a still, and alcohol vapour passed continuously into th mixture. The ensuing vapour, a mixture of ether, alcohol, and water, is scrubbed with sodium hydroxide to remove the sulphur dioxide and passed through a fractionating column from the top of which ether and alcohol come off as vapours. This is treated with alkaline permanganate, dried over calcium chloride, and distilled.

Table 1: Properties of Some Inhalation Anaesthetics

Anaesthetic	Oil/gas Coeff.	Molecular weight	Boiling Point (°C.)	Vapour Pressure at 20°C.	Liquid Density	Oil Water Solubility	Limits of Flammability (Per cent) a = in air; b = in O_2	Vapour Concentration for Anaesthesia (vol/per cent)	Minimal Alveolar Concentration for Anaesthesia (vol per cent)	Blood concentration for Anaesthesia (mg per cent)
Diethyl ether C_2H_5 C_2H_5	12.1	74	35	442		3.2	a. 1.85-36.5 b. 2-82	3-20 4	3.04	50-150 30-40
Divinyl ether C_2H_3 C_2H_3	.41	70	28.3	553	0.7	41.3	a. 1.7-27 b. 1.8-85	7-23 0.2-2	17.5	2.5-17 6-12
		42	-34	—	—	39	a. 2.4-10.3 b. 2.4	0.5-2 3-4.5		25-70 20-30
Cyclopropane C_3H_6	9.15	131	87.5	60	1.47	400	a. Non-flammable b. 10-64	4 50-80 0.5-2	— 188 0.87 (vol. per cent)	20-30 23-30
Trichloroethylene C_2HCl_3	7.32	119	61	160	1.49	100	Non-flammable	3-8 Up to 4	6.0 0.230	4-35 17-38
Chloroform $CHCl_3$		64.5	12.2	—	0.9	—	a. 4-14; b. 4- 67	— —	06-1.68 1.3	— —
Ethyl chloride C_2H_5Cl		72	35.8	428	0.76	45	a. 2.1 (lower limit) Non-flammable			
Ethyl-vinyl ether C_2H_5 C_2H_3	.46	44	-89	—	1.2	2.2	Non-flammable			
Nitrous oxide (N_2O)	2.3	197	50	243	1.86	330	a. 4.2; b. 4 Non-flammable			
Halothane $CF_3CHClBr$	1.57 13.0	126	42	—	1.13	94	Non-flammable			
Fluroxene $CF_3CH_2-O-CH=CH_2$	19.1 1.4	165	104.8	23	1.42	400	Non-inflammable			
Methoxyflurane $CHCl_2CF_2OCH_3$	0.69 0.42	—	56.5	184	1.52	98				
Enflurane		—	48.5	250	1.52	98				
Isoflurane			58.5	160						
Sevoflurane			22.8	664						
Desflurane										

Physical Properties

Colourless, volatile liquid of molecular weight 74, and specific gravity of 0.719. Boiling-point 35°C; saturated vapour pressure at 20°C is 442 mm. Hg; specific gravity of vapour 2.6 (i.e., it is two-and-a-half times heavier than air). Oil/water solubility ratio 3: 2. Blood/gas partition coefficient 15.0. Minimal alveolar concentration for anaesthesia is 3.04. Ether vapour is inflammable in air between 1.83 per cent and 36.5 per cent. Explosive in oxygen between 2-82 percent.

Chemical Properties

Relatively inert. May contain acetaldehyde and ether peroxide as impurities, due to decomposition, which is favoured by air, light, and heat and retarded by copper, iron, mercury, diphenylamine, and hydroquinone. Thus ether should be stored in dark cool places. Peroxides are probably the first impurities to develop in ether. They form within 6 months and persist for a year or more. Old ether contains fewer peroxides because aldehydes are then being formed. The greater the peroxide content, the less potent is the ether as an anaesthetic. Peroxides shown to be present if a yellow colour develops on addition of potassium iodide (shake 10 mL. ether with 10 per cent neutral potassium iodide; allow the mixture to remain in corked container in dark for 30 minute.; yellow colour in ether layer indicates liberation of iodine by peroxides.) Aldehydes in ether will cause Nessler's solution to turn turbid or yellow. (20 mL. of ether shaken) with 3 mL of reagent; two layers allowed to form; yellow colour in aqueous layer indicates presence of aldehydes).

It is largely unaltered in the body, 85 per cent to 90 per cent being eliminated by the lungs. The rate of elimination depends on the tidal exchange and blood-flow and can be expedited by heperventilation.

Pharmacology: Mercaptan–fishy smell. Toxic: 03%.

Circulatory System: Heart rate is increased at first due to:

(1) Catecholamines liberated; (2) Sympathetic stimulation; and (3) Vagal depression. Later, the heart rate is relatively unchanged. A light plane of anaesthesia causes vasoconstriction and a deep one vasodilatation, both effects on the vasomotor centre. Return of consciousness causes an increase of tone to a level greater than the original tone—hence the pallor.

Blood Pressure

If level of anaesthesia is below plane 2, a fall takes place after the first half-hour and is progressive, due to depression of smooth muscle in vessel walls; depression of skeletal muscle and consequent lack of support to circulation, reduced cardiac output, and depression of the vasomotor centre. There is peripheral vasodilatation, especially of face and head: the effect of this on the meningeal and cerebral vessels is to raise the cerebrospinal fluid pressure. But forearm vasoconstriction occurs due to liberation of noradrenaline. In deeper planes the vasomotor centre is paralysed so that peripheral vasodilatation is another cause of reduced blood pressure.

A functioning sympathetic nervous system is essential for the maintenance of blood pressure at normal levels during ether anaesthesia. Ether normally produces an increase in sympathoadrenal activity. The concentration of noradrenaline is substantially and consistently increased in deep anaesthesia and there appears to be some correlation between the levels and clinical signs such as increases in respiratory rate and volume and the degree of pupillary dilatation. There is also a significant relationship between plasma noradrenaline level and decrease in limb blood-flow with increased vascular resistance.

Respiratory System

Respiratory movements first increase due to mildly stimulating effects of ether vapour on the tracheobronchial mucosa and stimulation of the respiratory centre. This effect may be masked when a barbiturate or opiate has been given. They later decreases as anaesthesia deepens and the respiratory rate may be greater than thirty a minute during maintenance. In light surgical anaesthesia with ether, the respiratory centre continues to respond to carbon dioxide and the blood tension of this gas remains within fairly normal limits. This is not so in deep planes. Salivary, but not bronchial, secretions are increased, while bronchial muscles are relaxed. Bronchial and upper respiratory cilia is not inhibited by ether vapour. Vapour is irritating, producing cough and laryngeal spasm and perhaps, reflex apnoea, if introduced too rapidly. Hence induction of anaesthesia should be gradual, starting with a low ether tension. The Hering-Breuer reflex is depressed in Stage III, Plain 2, but in Plane 1 the reflex inhibition of inspiration on increasing intrabronchial pressure lasts 5 to 10 seconds. Useful in patients with tendency to bronchospasm and emphysema. Possible explanations[1] of the stimulating effect of ether on respiration include: (1) Direct stimulation of respiratory centre. (2) Stimulation of receptors in the lower respiratory tract. (3) Stimulation of pulmonary stretch receptors (similar to effect of trichloroethylene). (4) Stimulation of extrapulmonary receptors (muscles and joints). (5) Rise of noradrenaline levels.

Central Nervous System

Induces analgesia followed by excitement and then anaesthesia. Medullary depression is late and precedes serious cardiac depression. Meningeal and cerebral vessels dilate—an undesirable state in neurosurgery. Pressure of cerebrospinal fluid rises. Ether clonus, an exaggerated response to stretch reflexes, is sometimes seen during light anaesthesia.

The Sympathetic Nervous System: Central stimulation, resulting in increase of plasma noradrenaline with which is associated: (1) Increase of heart rate. (2) Increased production of glycogen and a raised blood-sugar level. (3) Contraction of spleen. (4) Dilatation of the gut and inhibition of its movements. (5) Bronchial dilatation. (6) Dilatation of coronary arteries. (7) Dilatation of pupils. (8) Decreased limb blood-flow with increased vascular resistance. (9) Increase in respiratory rate.

The Parasympathetic System: Central depression.

Alimentary System: Nausea and vomiting occur in more than 50 per cent of patients after ether anaesthesia. However, after use in minimal concentrations (2 to 3 per cent) in air with muscle relaxants for major surgery, no significant difference was found in the incidence of postoperative vomiting compared with other methods. Salivary glands are stimulated during induction and depressed later.

Gastrointestinal atony is produced in deep anaesthesia and postoperatively is more marked in the small than in the large bowel. This is due to stimulation of sympathetic nerves and atony of plain muscle. Liver function decreased but is restored to normal within twenty-four hours. Ether depresses the secretion of bile and bile salts.

The Urinary System: Urinary flow is diminished because of reduction in plasma volume and renal vascular constriction, a neurogenic effect, which soon passes off when anaesthesia is stopped.

In normal kidneys there is slight reduction of renal function, and this is greatly increased in cases of nephritis, and is not mediated through the posterior part of the pituitary. Both ether and cyclopropane cause renal vascular constriction.

The Pregnant Uterus: Movements inhibited, so that in deep anaesthesia relaxation is good. Ether passes the placental barrier and soon reaches the same concentration in foetal blood as in maternal blood. The oxygen-carrying capacity of the foetal blood is not altered.

Metabolism: Reduction in plasma bicarbonate and pH of blood and increase in blood carbon dioxide in deep planes. The explanation is probably that in deep ether anaesthesia there is overall depression of the respiratory centre which allows increase in alveolar and hence blood carbon dioxide, and this further depresses the respiratory centre. The importance of adequate ventilation follows, manually assisted, if necessary. Alterations in acid-base equilibrium are usually due to alterations in ventilation. Ketone bodies may appear and may be excreted in the urine. Metabolic acidosis is likely to occur in infants, or when disease causes depressed lactic acid metabolism (cirrhosis of the liver, Cushing's disease). Hyperglycaemia is common and blood-sugar levels may be increased two or threefold. One hour of surgical ether anaesthesia lowers the liver glycogen by 50 per cent. It is due to stimulation, arising from the midbrain, via sympathetic nerves to adrenal glands, causing mobilization of glycogen through extra secretion of adrenaline. If nerves to adrenals are paralysed no hyperglycaemia is produced by ether. Barbiturate (pentobarbitone) premedication inhibits this hyperglycaemia; morphine does not. After long periods of ether anaesthesia there are no microscopic changes in the liver.

Advantages of Ether
1. It is relatively non-toxic and would appear to upset the patient clinically less than biochemical investigation would suggest.
2. It will produce excellent relaxation without undue respiratory depression.
3. Respiratory depression is not accompanied by serious cardiac damage—in the absence of hypoxia. Artificial respiration will usually overcome the effects of temporary overdosage.
4. The ether is a very safe anaesthetic. For the unskilled anaesthetist dealing with the unfit patient it has a lot to commend it.

Light Ether Analgesia: The advantages of light ether narcosis have been pointed out by Artusio, who separated the first stage into three planes, in the deepest of which he claims to produce true analgesia with a fully conscious and co-operative patient. The technique is recommended by its originator for cardiac surgery.

Disadvantages of Ether
1. Its tendency to cause mucus secretion from the upper airway.
2. Its tendency to upset the body chemistry.
3. Its tendency to cause albuminuria.
4. Its tendency to explode when in contact with sparks, flames, and hot surfaces in the presence of oxygen or nitrous oxide.

The concentration of ether in the blood ranges from 100 to 170 mg per cent, from light anaesthesia to respiratory failure.

The inspiratory ether concentration necessary for laparotomy ranges from 6.1 to 13.7 vol per cent. Light anaesthesia can be maintained by 3 to 6 per cent (25 to 50 mm. Hg partial pressure) in inspired mixture.

Ether Convulsions: These have been reported since 1926. The classic case is the feverish child with a perforated appendix, on a hot day, who receives atropine premedication and ether anaesthesia, with the surgeon continually requesting more relaxation. They are not due exclusively to ether and may occur during overdosage of ether; impurities in ether; excessive temperature of the patient due either to his own illness or to the warmth and humidity of the operating theatre; carbon dioxide excess; carbon dioxide lack; sepsis; calcium deficiency; cerebral congestion; atropine excess; a specific streptococcus producing a neurotoxin, situated in the nasopharynx. Many of the convulsions occur in children and young adults. Death may follow from anoxia.
Convulsions give rise to hypoxia due to spasm of laryngeal and chest wall muscles, exhaustion & hyperpyrexia.

CLINICAL SIGNS OF ANAESTHESIA

Guedel developed his classic table of the signs of anaesthesia with division, into stages and planes, using open ether, that a really detailed system became generally accepted.

The Stages of Anaesthesia (using volatile agents, especially ether) (Fig. 1)

First Stage—Analgesia: From beginning of induction to loss of consciousness. Also known as 'the stage of disorientation'. Artusio[1] has subdivided this stage into three planes in the deepest of which true analgesia is said to coexist with consciousness and co-operation from the patient. These planes are apparent during recovery from deeper stages of anaesthesia.

Second Stage—Excitement of Uninhibited Response: From loss of consciousness to onset of automatic breathing. There may be struggling, breath-holding, vomiting, coughing, swallowing, etc. Can be minimized by adequate pre-medication, psychological preparation of the patient, quiet surroundings, and rapid smooth induction, Emergence delirium may occur during recovery from anaesthesia, especially with cyclopropane.

Third Stage—Surgical Anaesthesia: From onset of automatic respiration to respiratory paralysis. Guedel divided it into four planes:

PLANE 1: From onset of automatic respiration to cessation of eyeball movement.
PLANE 2: From cessation of eyeball movement to commencement of intercostal paralysis.
PLANE 3: From commencement to completion of intercostal paralysis.
PLANE 4: From complete intercostal paralysis to diaphragmatic paralysis.

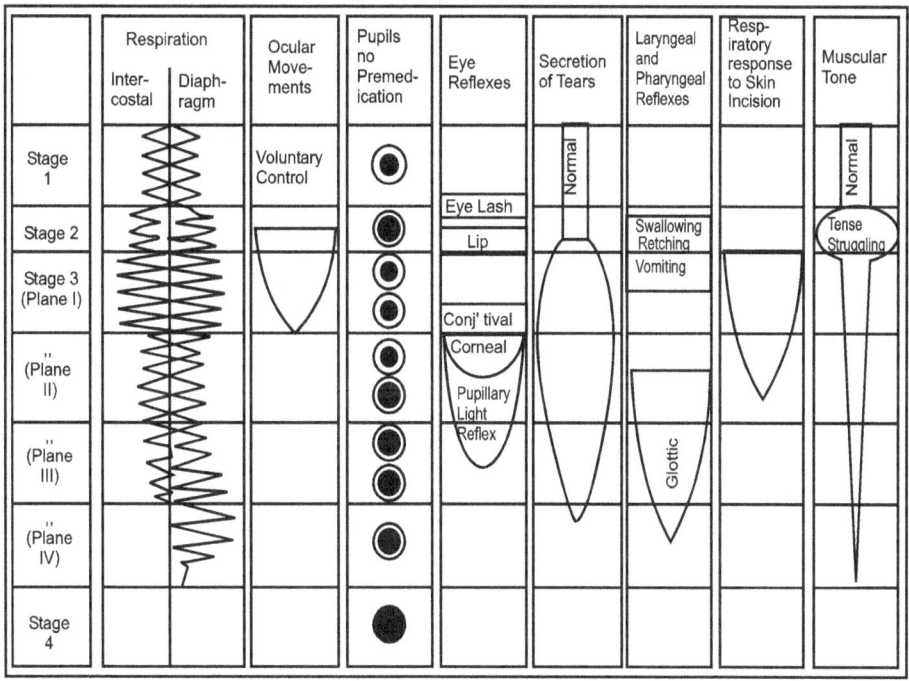

Fig. 1: The levels of disappearance of reflexes (after Guedel)

Ethyl chloride (C_2H_5Cl)

Ethylchloride is a highly volatile liquid with B.P. 2.5°C. S.V.P. 1.3 ATM at 20°C, Mol Wt. 64. SG = 2.2

Supplied in a pure form for general anaesthesia and in a less pure form, with a smaller nozzle, for local analgesia. Eau-de-Cologne is added to some brands to disguise the odour. The pressure of ethylchloride in its glass container is 30 to 40 mm. Hg above atmospheric pressure, cannot be used in closed circuits, as it is hydrolysed by the soda lime. Eliminated unchanged from lungs.

Pharmacology: Action on the central nervous system similar to that of the other volatile anaesthetics. Anaesthetic concentration is 3 to 4.5 vols per cent in inhaled gases. Blood concentration during anaesthesia ranges from 20 to 30 mg per cent. The safety margin is small owing to its volatility and relatively low blood/gas partition coefficient (2.0).

Cardiovascular System: Heart rate first decreases, a vagus effect; later increases. The initial vagal stimulation necessitates that atropine should always be used as premedication. The heart muscle is directly depressed and ventricular fibrillation has been reported, though this is extremely rare. Adrenaline may increase myocadial irritability. The blood pressure is decreased due to depression of vasomotor centre.

Respiratory System: The respiratory centre is first stimulated, later depressed. The stage of hyperpnoea is sometimes taken advantage to pass a blind nasal tube. Apnoea may occur in deeper planes. The drug should then be withdrawn and the lungs ventilated with air or oxygen to encourage elimination of the agent. Only slightly irritating to mucous membranes.

Muscular System : Nausea and vomiting are frequent after anaesthesia.

Signs of Anaesthesia : Induction may be stormy, but gives way in a matter of seconds to the regular breathing and muscular relaxation of surgical anaesthesia. Breathing is deeper than normal and becomes stertorous before overdosage causes it to become progressively shallower. If mask is removed after a few stertorous respirations when amplitude of breathing is maximal, about one minute of anaesthesia will result, followed by a shorter period of analgesia.

Advantages of Ethylchloride
1. Portability.
2. Rapid induction and recovery.
3. Economy.
4. Will not explode, though it burns.

Disadvantages
1. Postoperative nausea and vomiting.
2. Extreme potency and hence potential danger.

Indications: Many anaesthetists believe that, because of its extreme potency, ethylchloride should never be used. The advent of halothane has lessened the indications for its use. Other anaesthetists use ethylchloride, with due care, for induction of anaesthesia in children prior to ether maintenance, or as a sole agent for short operations.

CHLOROFORM [CHCL$_3$]

Prepared in 1831 by Justus von Leibg (1803 to 1873) in Germany, by Samuel Guthrie (1782 to 1848) in the US and by Eugene Soubeiran (1793 to 1858) in France. It was known as 'chloric ether', 'Dutch liquid', 'buchloric ether.'

Its high cardiac toxicity lead to its withdrawl from use, inspite of positive reports of Ist and IInd Chloroform Commissions in Hyderabad.

THE FLURINATED HYDROCARBONS

This group was known to be highly stable volatile and non-inflammable. In these compounds the fluorine atoms have a strong chemical bond with the carbon atoms. The result is that the fluorine atom is quite unreactive, particularly when the compound contains a CF_2 on CF_3 grouping. They are unlikely to interfere with body metabolism because of their high chemical stability and hence would tend to have low toxicity (Fig 2).

Those with low boiling points produce convulsive movements; that the potency increased as the boiling point rose yet recovery time became more prolonged and that substitution of bromine atom in the fluorohydro carbon not only, increased potency but also appeared to improve the safety margin. The inclusion of several halogen atoms in a compound confers inflammability in clinical range.

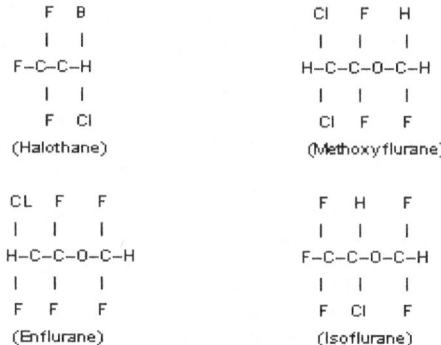

Fig. 2 : Composition of florinated hydrocarbons

HALOTHANE

Introduction

It was prepared and examined by Raventos. It was introduced into clinical anaesthesia by John Stone and Bryce-Smith and O Brien.

Physical Properties

    a. It is a heavy, colourless liquid with a sweat smell somewhat resembling chloroform. It contains 0.01% of thymol for stability.
    b. It does not react with soda lime and one of the contaminants, is betene in a concentration of 0.001%.
    c. The vapour pressure of halothane is 24 mmHg at 20°C. Hence it is very suitable for vaporisation in a bubble through or temperature and flow controlled vaporiser.
    d. It's readily soluble in rubber and less so in polyethylene.
    e. It can be estimated by gas chromatography or by infrared or by ultraviolet light.

Pharmacology

MAC

MAC value of halothane is 0.8 but is reduced to about 0.3 when N_2O 70% is added as a carrier gas.

Uptake and Distribution

It has a blood solubility coefficient of 2.3. Because it is relatively insoluble in blood it is not taken up very rapidly from alveoli. Hence the alveolar concentration can soon approach the inspired concentration. Alveolar concentration is same as of brain concentration and hence induction of anaesthesia is rapid. This first goes to the organs of rich blood supply like heart and brain. Resting muscle and fat have a much poorer blood supply so that they receive their quota of halothane long after the tension in alveoli and brain have reached equilibrium. 1% inspired concentration given to a patient, will take 5 days for the concentration in the alveoli to rise to this level. One of the principal reasons for the prolonged uptake of halothane by the body is the remarkable capacity of fat to absorb it.

Metabolism

About 12% of inspired halothane is metabolised by liver microsomes and resulting products are excreted in urine[8]. Halothane undergoes both oxidation and dehalogenation to form trifluoracetic acid as well as chloride and bromide radicals. This metabolism may be stimulated by barbiturates. Chronic halothane exposure can impair liver cell functional.

Actions

1. **On respiration:** Halothane is a respiratory depressant, more so in presence of narcotic premedication. In view of respiratory depression, it is advisable occasionally to assist the ventilation whenever spontaneous respiration is present. At least 30% oxygen should always be present in the inspired mixture. Halothane may be accidentally injected intravenously in which case severe pulmonary lesions leading to death occur.

2. **On Heart:** The cardiac contractile force was diminished; stroke volume and cardiac output were reduced despite an increased venous pressure. The heart rate and arterial pressure were also reduced[9]. There is increased incidence of arrythmias due to :
   - Decreases automaticity of SA node, thereby favouring the emergence of alternative pacemakers.
   - Slows myocardial conductions which favours the re-entry of cardiac impulse.
   - Halothane interacts with adrenaline, thus increasing incidence of arrythmia.
   Halothane may also interact with calcium channel blockers more so with intravenous route. It also has a protective effect in myocardial ischaemia if it's commenced before ischaemia occurs and also improves recovery post ischaemia. The baro receptors reflex is completly inhibited at 1.1% end tidal concentration of halothane.

3. **On peripheral circulation:** There is a persistent vasodilatation produced by halothane on vessels of skin and muscle along with a fall in both the arterial pressure and vascular resistance. Halothane does not have a direct action on the vessel itself but acts rather by blocking the action of noradrenaline.

4. **On kidney and liver:** Halothane causes a decrease in renal flow probably related to a fall in glomerular filtration rate and a reduction in ADH release. It also leads to a fall in hepatic blood flow.

5. **On uterus:** Halothane anaesthesia relaxes uterine muscle in direct relation to the depth of anaesthesia due to direct stimulation of the adrenergic -receptors of uterus. There are possible dangers of increased bleeding from the uterus after the use of halothane.

6. **On GIT**: In anaesthestic concentrations, halothane depresses the motility of jejunum, colon and stomach. It's also capable of antagnising the contractions produced by the parenteral administration of neostigmine.
7. **On skeletal muscles**: Halothane has minimal neuromuscular blocking action but potentiates the action of the nondepolarising agents.
8. **On cerebral blood flow**: CBF is increased and cerebral vascular resistance decreased during halothane anaesthesia. Headache may follow halothane anaesthesia.
9. **Others**: Intense muscle spasms occasionally observed in early postoperative period. They are called 'Halothane shakes' may be due to vasodilatory action of drug. Sometimes it interferes with mitosis in cells. The drug is most effective in reducing shivering is pethidine. Oxygen consumption is significantly increased and hypoxaemia may result. There is significant heat loss during anaesthesia and the cutaneous vasodilatation may occur.

Toxicity

A major problem associated with the use of halothane is hepatotoxicity. Out of the two pathways of halothane metabolism, the reductive pathway is favoured in low oxygen tension conditions leading to production of toxic metabolite,thus causing rise of liver enzymes. Another form is hepatic necrosis which is immune mediated. Hence its advised that halothane administration should not be repeated within 3 months. The metabolite TFA halide bind is to hepatocytes, creating neoantigens and thereby exciting an autoimmune response against hepatocyte. Tests like immunoblotting assay and ELISA are used to detect this.

Halothane decomposes on contact with soda lime to CF_2 CCI Br which is nephrotoxic.

It also triggers malignant hyperthermia where in there is defect in their skeletal muscle that makes them susceptible to massive release of intracellular calcium from sarcoplasmic reticulum (SR) of skeletal muscle on exposure to halothane. There is increased metabolism of muscle leading to a rise of temperature over 2°C per hour and serious biochemical derangement. Rhabdomyolysis with hyperkalaemia occurs. Management includes supportive measures, active cooling and use of muscle relaxant dantrolene which inhibits release of calcium for SR.

ENFLURANE

Introduction

It's one of the 700 compounds produced by RC Terell of Ohio medical products. It was first tested in man in 1966. A major potential advantage of enflurane is its much more stability in the body than other agents.

Physical Properties

- Clear, colourless, non-inflammable liquid.
- Specific gravity 1.52 at 25°C.
- Boiling point 56.5°
- Vapour pressure 184 mmHg at 20°C.
- It contains no chemical stabilisers and is non-corrosive and may be stored in clear glass.
- It's entirely compatible with soda lime and has pleasant ethereal smell.
- Blood/gas solubility coefficient is 191 at 37°C which explains swift induction and emergence.
- Rate of metabolism is 1/5th of halothane and thus has greater chemical stability which reduces toxicity of metabolities [10].

Pharmacology

- MAC: MAC of enflurane is 1.68 in young adults and decreases to 0.6% when 70% N_2O is added as a carrier gas.
- Uptake and distribution: The blood/gas solubility is 1.8 which signifies that it's relatively insoluble in blood. Thus relatively rapid induction and emergence is expected.

Action

1. **On respiratory system:** It's non-irritant to the respiratory tract with no excessive salivation but high concentrations may cause breath holding coughing and even laryngospasm. Enflurane has highest 'Apnoea index' (ratio of apnoea dose to anaesthetic dose) compared to other agents. Halothane and enflurane produce broncho-dilatation and hence advised to be used for COPD patients. They diminished airflow resistance by substantial reduction in broncho motor tone.
2. **On cardiovascular system:** At 1MAC it reduces cardiac output, arterial pressure, systemic vascular resistance and rate of rise of pressure in aorta. But no further drops after rising MAC above 1.5 in cardiac output is seen. It has been seen to potentiate the hypotensive effects of sodium nitroprusside and fentanyl. It depresses the contractility of cardiac muscle by inhibition of uptake of calcium ions by the sarcoplasmic reticulum of cardiac muscle. They prolong conduction time at AV node but enflurane has sparing effect on Purkinje system, thus has fewer arrthymias.
3. **On central nervous system:** Change in EEG pattern is seen with increasing depth of anaesthesia characterised by high voltage, high frequency spike and one activity on frank seizure activity. Abnormal neuromuscular activity in form of twitching, clonus, or stiffness of extremities is seen. Cerebral blood flow is unchanged or reduced by enflurane anaesthesia. Cerebral oxygen consumption ($CMRO_2$) decreases markedly with low dose of enflurane anaesthesia.
4. **In obstetrics:** Low dose enflurane (0.5 to 1%) has been used to supplement anaesthesia in obstetric surgery; there was no awareness or factual recall. It depresses contractions and tone of gravid and non-gravid myometrium. Blood loss is decreased with enflurane anaesthesia.
5. **On skeletal muscle:** It has intrinsic muscle relax property by depression of post synaptic responses to acetylcholine thus inhibiting end plate depolarisation. All patients anaesthetised with volatile anaesthetics require less muscle relaxation due to block of neuromuscular transmission.

Toxicity

It results in formation of TFA which cause hepatotoxicity. Concentrations of fluoride greater than 50 mmol/L are associated with renal impairment. Characterized by serum hypernatremia, urinary hyposomolarity and vasopressin resistant polyuria. Production of carbon monoxide when enflurane is exposed to soda lime or baralyme is another problem [12]. This happens mainly when soda lime is dried out. Normal water content is 15% carbon monoxide production is negligible above 4.8%. This is greater with baralyme. Uptake of fluroide ion from serum to bone is as important as excretion in urine as this accounts for almost half the fluroide load. More important in renal dysfunction as greater amounts of fluoride enter bone thus protecting the kidney from prolonged exposure.

ISOFLURANE

Introduction

It was first produced in 1968 by Dr. RC Terell as one of the 700 compounds he produced. It was approved for clinical use in USA in 1979 and in UK by 1983.

Physical Properties
- Clear, colourless, non-inflammable liquid.
- Specific gravity 1.52 at 25°C.
- Boiling point 48.5°C.
- Vapour pressure of 250 mmHg at 20°C.
- Contains no chemical stabilizers and is non-corrosive and is stored in clear glass.
- Stable in warm soda lime and has slightly pungent ethereal smell.
- Blood/ gas solubility 1.4 at 37°C.
- Greater chemical stability, less production of metabolities and less toxicity.

Pharmacology
- **MAC:** MAC is 1.3% in young adults, decreased to 1% in elderly; addition of 70% N_2O decreases MAC to 0.6 in young and to 0.4% in elderly patients[13].
- **Uptake and Distribution :** Blood/gas coefficient of this drug is 1.4 and hence is faster acting. Oil/gas coefficient is 98 and hence is a weak anaesthetic. Vapour pressure of 250 mmHg makes it possible to deliver whatever concentration is required from the same vaporisers used for halothane. Awakening is predictably rapid. The pungent odour, through breath holding and coughing, limit the speed of induction of anaesthesia. This can be overcome by premedicant and step-by step increments in inspired concentration of 0.5% every 5 breaths to a maximum of 4%. It's only slightly soluble in materials used for construction of anaesthetic circuits.

Actions
1. **On respiratory system:** It's a potent respiratory depressant. At 1% MAC, spontaneous ventilation in unstimulated patients is reduced so that $PaCO_2$ is 50 mmHg; at 15% it is 65 mmHg and ventilatory response to imposed increases in $PaCO_2$ progressively and linearly approach at about 2.0 MAC. Ventilatory responses to hypoxia are markedly reduced by isoflurane at 0.1 MAC and virtually disappear at 1 MAC.
2. **On cardiovascular system:** It has a direct myocardial depressant effect. Arterial blood pressure and total peripheral vascular resistance are reduced in a dose-related manner. Decrease in blood pressure is due to vasodilation as a result of direct relaxation of vascular smooth muscle, by enhanced formation of cyclic adenosine-5-monophosphate in regional circulations of skin, muscle, brain, heart and splanchnic. Blood flow to muscle is particularly enhanced by 2 to 3 fold. There appears to be a wide margin of cardiovascular safety with isoflurane; the cardiac index (ratio of dose producing cardiac arrest versus MAC) is 5.7. Central venous oxygen saturation increases and base excess changes are minimal. It does not affect heart rhythm and dysrythmias following injection of adrenaline are less likely than halothane.
3. **On central nervous system:** It causes a dose related depression, substantial changes occur between 0.25 and 0.5 MAC and amnesia at 0.25. It doesn't have convulsive activity or impair intracellular functions. It does not increase cerebral blood flow at 0.6 to 1.1 MAC, but it doubles at 1.6 MAC. Cerebral metabolism is decreased which may lead to a decrease in blood flow, useful in conditions of increased ICP.
4. **Neuromuscular effects:** It can produce adequate muscle relaxation for most surgical manoeuvre; but for abdominal procedures it is desirable to use muscle relaxant drugs to avoid undesirable effects of prolonged inhalation of concentrations in excess of 1.0 MAC. It enhances the action of nondepolarizing muscle relaxants.

Metabolism and Toxicity

Hepatotoxicity has been noticed with isoflurane anaesthesia. The mechanism of toxicity is probably a result of TFA metabolite forming neoantigens. Fluoride ions are also produced by isoflurane metabolism, but in clinically insignificant amounts because of low rate of metabolism. There is no evidence of nephrotoxicity. It is a trigger for malignant hyperthermia in susceptible patients. There is no evidence of mutagenicity, teratogenicity and carcinogenicity.

SEVOFLURANE

Introduction

It was first synthesized in late 1960 at Baxter-Travenol Laboratory by RF Wallin and Coworkers. First used in humans in 1981, but stopped and banned due to two drawbacks' (Fig 13.3) i.e., metabolism results in production of potentially significant levels of fluoride ions and is chemically unstable in presence of soda lime. Then a Japanese firm, Maruishi pharmaceuticals (Osaka) in 1990 got it approved and its use started.

Physical Properties

- Contains no chlorine or bromine ions so does not have effect on ozone layer.
- Colourless, noninflammable and liquid.
- Boiling point of 58.5°C and not unpleasant.
- Vapour pressure 160 mmHg at 20°C.
- Less soluble in rubber and plastic.
- MAC 3.3 in neonates decrease to 1.48 in elderly [15].

Pharmacology

- **Uptake and distribution**: It has blood/gas coefficient of 0.69 which is half of isoflurane and quarter of halothane. Induction and recovery should, therefore, be more rapid. Anaesthetic concentrations are rapidly achieved. Sevoflurane is primarily exerted through the lung; although a small amount is metabolized. The proportion metabolized has been estimated at between 1.6% and 4.9%.
- **Metabolism**: Metabolism occurs in liver, catalyzed by the cytochrome P 450 2E1 enzyme. It is broken down into inorganic fluoride ions and the organic fluoride metabolite hexa- fluoroisopropanol (HFIP). HFIP is conjugated with glucuronic acid to form HFIP glucuroide, which is excreted by kidneys. No evidence of toxicity associated with HFIP [16].

Actions

1. **On central nervous system**: It causes similar dose dependent changes in EEG. There is evidence of EEG changes consistent with seizure activity in a non– epileptic patient under deep sevoflurane anaesthesia and also a report of tonic clonic seizure like movements in a patient recovering from sevoflurane anaesthesia. Although mean arterial pressure of cerebral perfusion pressure are well maintained. It causes slight increase in ICP in normocapnic patients.
2. **On respiratory system**: It is quite pleasant to inhale and has no irritant effect on the airway. This combined with its low blood/gas solubility makes it very suitable for inhalational induction. It's a respiratory depressant causing a reduction in minute ventilation. Tidal volume is reduced and respiratory rate is increased. The ventilatory response to CO_2 is depressed to a slightly greater degree than with halothane and 0.1 MAC causes a 30 to 40% depression of the ventilatory response to hypoxia. It's also effective as a bronchodilator.
3. **On cardiovascular effects**: It has minimal effect on heart rate. It can produce direct myocardial depression through effect on calcium channels. It causes a dose dependent depression of cardiac output and a reduction in systemic vascular resistance. It does not

sensitize the myocardium to epinephrine. It is a coronary vasodilator. It also protects against some of the metabolic changes associated with myocardial ischaemia.

4. **Neuromuscular effects:** It produces a dose dependent muscle relaxation. At deeper levels of anaesthesia, it provides sufficient relaxation to allow tracheal intubation.

Toxicity

Metabolism of sevoflurane results in the production of inorganic fluoride ions and HFIP. Although serum inorganic fluoride levels are greater than 50 mol/L a degradation product called compound A is formed when sevoflurane is exposed to soda lime or baralyme due to its absorption. Compounds A–E are formed out of which compound A causes lung and renal damage. The lower the flow in a circle system, the higher will be the concentration of compound A, the addition of water to soda–lime and the use of partially exhausted soda–lime seems to reduce the production of compound during low fluoride anaesthesia. Despite its relatively high metabolism, sevoflurane does not appear to be hepatotoxic. As with other volatile agents, sevoflurane should be avoided in patients susceptible to malignant hyperthermia.

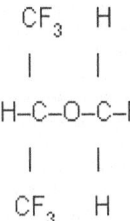

Fig 13.3 : Structure of Sevoflurance

DESFLURANE

Introduction

It was another one in the series of 700 compounds produced by Dr. Ross Terrell.

Physical Properties

- It's a fluorinated methyl ethyl ether.
- It contains no chlorine or bromine ions and hence does not deplete ozone layers.
- Pungent odor which makes it irritating and unpleasant to inhale.
- Boiling point 22.8°C.
- Vapour pressure 664 mmHg at 20°C and hence it can't be administered using a standard vaporizer. A new vaporizer has been developed to administer this agent which converts it into agas by heating it to a constant temperature and then maintaining it at a constant pressure. This vaporizer needs an external power source.

Pharmacology

Uptake and Distribution

It has lowest blood/gas solubility coefficient of 0.42. Hence it has fastest induction and recovery. The elimination is also faster; which is almost exclusively through the lungs, with metabolism by liver estimated to be less than 0.02%. Increased serum on urine fluoride levels have not been seen.

MAC: MAC of desflurane is 4.58% to 7.25%[17]. depending on stimulus used; MAC decreases with increasing age, MAC is reduced by nitrous oxide.

Actions

1. **On central nervous system:** It produces a dose dependent suppression of EEG. No evidence of any epileptiform activity. It causes dose dependent cerebral vasodilation and a dose dependent reduction in cerebral metabolism. It increases lumbar CSF pressure in normocapnic patients without an intracranial mass lesion.
2. **On respiratory system:** It is unsuitable for inhalation induction as it is extremely irritant to the airway. Concentrations > 6% cause coughing, breath holding and laryngospasm. It is a potent respiratory depressant. It causes a dose dependent decrease in tidal volume and an increase in respiratory rate. It causes concentration dependent bronchodilation.
3. **On cardiovascular system:** It causes a dose dependent tachycardia associated with a depression in myocardial contractility and a decrease in SVR resulting from peripheral vasodilation. It's a direct coronary vasodilator and decreases overall cardiac work. A rapid increase in the concentration of desflurane to greater than 1MAC will cause increase in heart rate and blood pressure.
4. **Neuromuscular effects:** It significantly depresses neuromuscular function. It reduces the force of contraction of the adductor pollicis muscle and increases the degree of tetanic fade. It can provide sufficient relaxation to allow tracheal intubation. It also potentiates the action of non depolarising muscle relaxants.

Toxicity

It has very low blood /gas and blood tissue solubility; is very stable and undergoes minimal metabolism. A very small amount of desflurane is metabolised with the production of TFA, which may interact with hepatic proteins and induce an immune response in susceptible patients. There is no evidence of renal toxicity even after prolonged exposure. It can act as a trigger agent for malignant hyperthermia.

BARBITURATES
BASIC PHARMACOLOGY
Chemistry and Formulation (Fig 4)

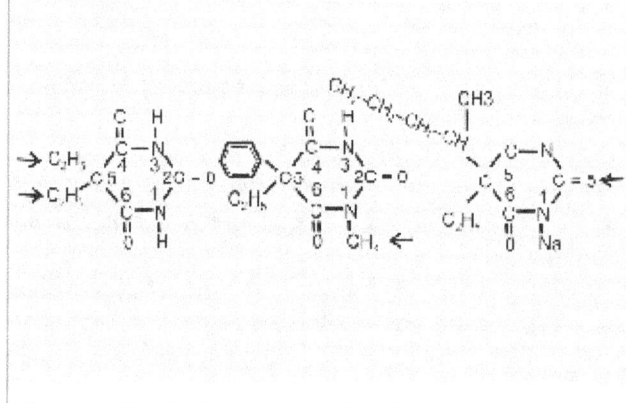

Fig. 13.4 : Chemical structure of activity relationship of barbiturates

The barbiturates are derivatives of barbituric acid (2, 4, 6 –Trioxohexahydropyrimidine) or it's 2-thio analogue. Also called cyclic uriede of malonic acid as it is synthesised from urea and malonic acid, barbituric acid is actually a pyrimidine nucleus [18]. Commonly used barbiturates are:
- Thiopental (5-ethyl-5- (1-methylbutyl)-2 thio– barbituric acid).
- Thiamylal (5-allyl-5-(1-methylbutyl)-2-thiobarbituric acid).
- Methohexital (methylated oxybarbiturate).

The sodium salts of these drugs which are mixed with 6% by weight anhydrous sodium carbonate are reconstituted with either water or 0.9% sodium chloride to produce 2.5%, 2.0%, 1/.0% solutions of thiopental, thiamylal and methohexital respectively. Buffering action of sodium carbonate in presence of atmospheric CO_2 maintains moderate alkalinity (pH 10–11) of barbiturate solutions. Properly reconstituted thiobarbiturate solutions are stable for 1 week, if refrigerated, while it is 6 weeks in case of methohexital [19].

Structure Activity Relationship

Hypnotic activity is introduced into the barbituric acid molecule by addition of side chains, especially if at least one of them is branched in position 5. The length of side chain in position 5 influences the potency and duration of action of the barbituric acid derivatives. Many barbiturates have asymmetric acid derivatives. Many bariburates have asymmetric carbon atoms in one of the side chains attached to carbon 5 of the barbiturate ring. The L-isomere of pertobarbital, secobarbital, thiopental and thiamylal are nearly twice as potent as the d-isomers despite their similar access to CNS. These barbiturates are marked as racemic mixture. Methohexital has 4 stereoisomers.

Mechanism of Action

The gama-aminobutyric acid ($GABA_A$) receptor complex is the most likely site of barbiturate action. GABA receptor is an oligomeric complex consisting of 5 subunits which assemble to form a chloride ion channel with a $GABA_A$ receptor, benzodiazepine, barbiturate, steroid and picrotoxin binding sites. Activation of $GABA_A$ receptor increases chloride conductance through the channel, hyperpolarizing and thereby reducing the excitability of the postsynaptic neurons [20]. They are also called ligand gated chloride ion channels.

Barbiturates both enhance and mimic the action of GABA. By binding of their receptor, they increase the rate of dissociation of GABA from its receptor and increase the duration of GABA activated chloride ion channel openings.

Pharmacokinetics and Pharmacodynamics

Thiopental directly rapidly mixes within a central blood pool and is distributed by blood flow and molecular diffusion throughout the tissues of the body according to their rate of perfusion, their affinity for drug and the relative concentrate of thiopental in tissues and blood. The highly perfused, relatively low volume tissues such as brain, equilibrate rapidly with the high early concentrations of thiopental in the blood, resulting in induction of anaesthesia. Thiopental concentration in the blood and highly perfused tissue then increase rapidly as the drug redistributes to the large reservoir of less well perfused lean tissue like muscle, thus terminating the effect of an induction dose. Despite to its high affinity for thiopental, adipose tissue takes up drug slowly because of its poor perfusion.

A real-time index of the effect of thiopental may be produced by bispectral index (BIS). It is a measure of hypnotic effect that is computed from EEG data and is reported as a value between 0 and 100. A patient maintained at a BIS of < 55 from the time of induction of anaesthesia with thiopental until maintenance anaesthetic concentrations are adequate, would have a small probability of awareness.

Clinical Pharmacology and Uses

1. **Night time hypnosis and premedication:** Pentobarbital and secobarbital provides night time drowsiness and premedication prior to surgery before benzodiazepines replaced them.
2. **Induction of general anaesthesia**
   (a) **Drugs and dosage:** Thiopental, thiamylal and methohexal, one can be injected IV to induce general anaesthesia and can also be used to maintain unconsciousness as the hypnotic component of a balanced anaesthetic technique or a total IV anaesthetic technique. They induce anaesthesia rapidly and pleasantly and are less expensive than propofol. When injected IV, this lipid soluble drugs act in one-arm brain circulation time and have their maximum effect in about one minute.
   An induction dose of 1.5 mg/kg of methohexital is equivalent to 4 mg/kg of thiopental, thus, methohexital appears to be about 2.7 times as potent.
   (b) **Injection complications:** There may be urticarial rash of the upper chest, neck and face that fades off after few minutes. Anaphylactoid reactions such as liver and facial oedema, bronchospasm and shock occur occasionally. Treatment of these reactions is symptomatic but should include 1 mL increments of 1: 10,000 epinephrine and IV fluids. Aminophylline can be given to treat bronchospasm. Incidence of pain on injection is 1 to 2% after thiopental and upto 5% after methohexital when injected into the small veins on the back of the hand or wrist essentially none when injected into larger veins. They are extravasated; pain, oedema and erythema ensue and reactions ranging from slight soreness to extensive tissue necrosis can occur locally.
   When injected intra arterially, intense arterial spasm results and excruciating pain can be felt from the injection site to the hand and fingers. The onset of pain and burning is immediate and can persist for hours. A range of symptoms from mild discomfort to gangrene and loss of tissue in hand can result. The pathological process is chemical endarteritis, which destroys the endo-thelium, subendothelial tissues which induces dilution of barbiturate, relieve spasm and prevent thrombosis. Injection of papaverine 40 to 80 mg in 10 to 20 mL of normal saline or 5 to 10 mL of 1% lidocaine or procaine into the artery may accomplish the first two objectives. Stellate ganglion block or brachial plexus block can relieve spasm. Heparin can be given to prevent thrombosis.
   (c) **Side effects during induction of anaesthesia :**
   Approximately 40% patients describe an onion or garlic taste between injection of thiopental and unconsciousness; more so in young patients. Also some mild muscular excitatory movements such as hypertonus, tremor/twitching and respiratory excitatory effects including cough and hiccup. Inadequate dose of induction can also evoke excitatory responses because inhibitory areas of brain are the first to be depressed.

Specific Organ Function Effects
1. **CNS Effects**
   - The barbiturates may be hyperalgesic in sub-anaesthetic concentration; exaggerating response to pain. The clinical signs include tachycardia, hypertension, diaphoresis, tearing and tachypnoea.
   - It induces a dose-related depression of EEG. The awake pattern progresses to higher amplitude and slower frequency and theta– waves until there is burst suppression and finally a flat EEG [20].
   - Dose-dependent depression of cerebral metabolism of oxygen i.e., $CMRO_2$ which reaches a maximum of 55 where the EEG becomes flat. There is parallel reduction of

CBF and ICF. This is particularly beneficial for patient with increased ICP. Cerebral perfusion pressure is not compromised as ICP increased more than mean arterial pressure. Thus, thiopental is an appropriate drug to induce anaesthesia for neurosurgery.
- Thiopental is also preferred for high-dose administration or prolonged use for neuroanaesthesia because patients have been reported to have epileptiform seizures after very high doses of methohexital.
- IV barbiturates are safe to use in ophthalmic procedures including those for open eye surgeries. IOP increased by 40% after an induction dose of thiopental or methohexital.

2. Respiratory effects
- These agents cause central respiratory depression, the nature and duration of which depend on the dose, rate of injection and type and dose of premedication; both rate and depth of breathing can be depressed until apnoea occurs.
- The responses to hypercarbia and hypoxaemia are depressed for longer times even if 2 mg/kg Thiopental dose is used.
- Thiopental depress the mucocilliary clearance of foreign material. They are safe in asthmatic patients; but they don't cause broncho dilation as ketamine does.

3. CVS effects
- Predominant effect is vasodilatation followed by pooling of blood in the periphery.
- Myocardial contractility is depressed due to interference with Ca^{2+} transport across myocardial cells and/or altering NO mechanism. They increase neuronal NO synthase activity.
- Cardiac output (CO) increases even though the HR increases via the only slightly depressed baro reflex mechanism.
- They cause dilatation of pulmonary vessels.
- No arrhythmia occur as long as hypoxia and hypercarbia are avoided.
- Also decrease sympathetic output from CNS and don't sensitize the heart to catecholamines.
- They increased HR which increased myocardial O_2 consumption.

4. GIT Renal and Hepatic Effects
- Hypoproteinaemia in patients with hepatic and renal diseases lead to a greater fraction of unbound thiopental than in healthy patients. Thus, in CRF patients, doses of thiopental should be injected at a slower rate and maintenance doses increased to 50–75%.
- They increase urine output as they increase blood flow to kidney, causing renal artery constriction and results in small increase in GFR and urinary solute secretion. Correcting hypotension and administering adequate IV fluids prevent renal effects of barbiturate induction from becoming a clinical problem.
- There is an increased ADH secretion from the pituitary which is yet controversial.

5. Metabolic Effects
- There is clinically a significant increase in blood glucose level and impairment of glucose tolerance test after thiopental injection.
- Heat loss results from vasodilatation caused by barbiturate induction of cutaneous and skeletal muscle vessels, leading to post–operative shivering.

6. Endocrine effects
- They increase cortisol plasma concentrations but do not prevent adrenocortical stimulation from stress of surgery.

7. Obstetric effects

- They neither depress nor increase the tone of gravid uterus. They are not harmful to the foetus when given for anaesthetic induction for caesarean section in doses upto 6 mg/kg.
- Safe delivery of foetus in caesarean section is possible if accomplished within 10 minutes after anaesthestic induction with thiopental.

Drug Interactions

Barbiturates when given to patients on CNS depressants drugs like ethanol, antihistamines isoniazid, methylphenidate and MAO inhibitors, cause greater CNS depression. Concomitant administration of 5–6 mg/kgaminophylline reduces both depth and duration of sedation after thiopental administration.

Recovery

It is rapid after many anaesthestic regimes that include IV barbarities. Clinically recovery is faster in infants < 14 years old. Ability to drive a motor vehicle is impaired for 8 hours after methohexital and 6 hours after thiopental. Hence advice is given not to drive for next 24 hours after general anaesthesia.

Postoperative Sequelae

- Venous sequelae include thrombosis and phlebitis which are confined to the area of the vein in close proximity to site of injection.
- Paralysis and death occur if barbiturates are given to patients with acute intermittent porphyria on variegate porphyria. This is owing to the induction of d-aminolevulinic acid synthetase which catalyzes the rate limiting step in the biosynthesis of porphyrins.

Other Uses

1. **Anticonvulsants:** They stop seizures abruptly in patients refractory to other anticonvulsant drugs but benzodiazepines (BZD) have replaced them [21]. They facilitate the action of GABA in prolonging hyperpolarization of the postsynaptic membrane. Other effects include altered membrane conductance of chloride ions and antagonism of glutaminergic and cholinergic excitation.
2. **Brain protection:** They increase cerebral metabolism in areas of high brain activity until EEG is flat. Possible mechanism are suppression of excitatory transmission by interfering with NO in vessels. It also protects the poorly perfused areas of the brain in patients with increased ICP.
3. **WADA Test:** A small dose of amobarbital can be injected into the carotid artery to lateralize cerebral speech dominance in neurosurgical patients. An alternative is injection of methohexital 3–5 mg after a 1` mg test dose.
4. **ECT:** Propofol resulted in shorter seizure duration, but BP was likely to rise above control values. Methohexital is preferable to thiopental as transient premature aterial and ventricular contraction occur less frequently after methohexital, whether or not atropine is used as premedication.

BENZODIAZEPINES

Physicochemical Properties

Three benzodiazepines receptor agonists are commonly used, i.e., midazolam, diazepam, lorazepam. These molecules are relatively small and are lipid soluble at physiological pH. Each mL of diazepam solution (5 mg) contains propylene glycol 0.4 mL, alcohol 0.1 mL, benzyl alcohol 0.015 mL and sodium benzoate/benzoic solution (pH 6.4 Lorazepam) (2–4 mg/mL) contains 0.18 mL polyethylene glycol with 2% benzyl alcohol as preservative.

Midazolam solution contains 1 on 5 mg/mL of midazolam with 0.8% sodium chloride and 0.01% disodium edetate, with 1% benzyl alcohol as preservative. The pH is adjusted to 3 with hydrochloric acid and sodium hydroxide. The imidazole ring of midazolam accounts for its stability in solution and rapid metabolism.

Metabolism

Biotransformation of benzodiazepines occurs in liver. Two principal pathways are either hepatic microsomal oxidation or glucuronide conjugation. Both midazolam and diazepam undergo oxidation– reduction or phase 1 reactions in the liver. The fused imidazole ring of midazolam is oxidized rapidly by the liver. There is greater hepatic clearance of midazolam compared with diazepam [22]. Habitual alcohol consumption increases clearance of midazolam. Diazepam has two active metabolites i.e., oxazepam and desmethyl diazepam both of which add to and prolong the drug's effects. These metabolities are rapidly conjugated and excreted in urine. The 1-hydroxymidazolam has 20–30% potency of midazolam. It is excreted by kidneys.

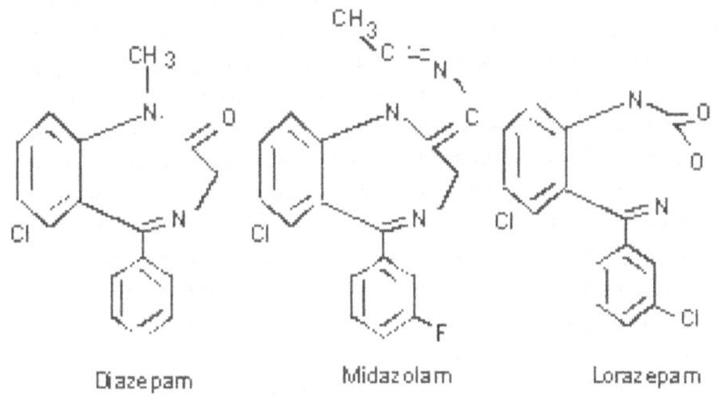

Fig.13.5 : Chemical Structures of Benzodiazepines

Lorazepam has five metabolites; but the principal one is conjugated to glucuronide which is inactive and water soluble.

Pharmacokinetics

The three benzodiazepines used in anaesthesia are classified as short-midazolam; intermediate-lorazepam; long-lasting diazepam, according to the metabolism and plasma clearance rate which is 6–11 mL/kg/min for midazolam, 0. to 1.8 mL/kg/min for lorazepam, 0.2 to 0.5 mL/kg/min for diazepam. Factors known to influence are age, gender, race, enzyme induction and hepatic and renal disease. All these drugs are affected by obesity.

Pharmacology

Midazolam is approximately 3–6 times and lorazepam is 5–10 times as potent as diazepam. All the actions are mediated at the benzodiazepine-gama-aminobutyric acid ($GABA_A$) receptor. These receptors are found in highest densities in the olfactory bulb, cerebral cortex, cerebellum, hippocampus, substantial nigra, and inferior colliculus with activation of $GABA_A$ receptor, gating of channel for chloride ions is triggered. The cell becomes hyperpolarized and, therefore, resistant to neuronal excitation. But hypnotic effects are mediated by the alterations in a potential dependent calcium ion flux [23]. Agonis alter the conformation of the $GABA_A$ receptors complex so that binding affinity for GABA is increased with the resultant opening of the chloride channels. Agonist and antagonist bind to a common area of the receptor by forming differing reversible bonds with the receptors. Antagonists occupy benzodiazepine receptors, but they produce no activity, therefore, block the actions of both the agonist and inverse agonists. Long term administration of benzodiazepines produces tolerance.

Actions
1. On central nervous system: They reduce the cerebral metabolic rate of oxygen consumption ($CMRO_2$) and cerebral blood flow (CBF). Midazolam, diazepam and lorazepam; all increase the seizure initiation threshold to local anaesthetics. They also cause a dose related protective effect against cerebral hypoxia. The protection afforded by midazolam is superior to that of diazepam but less than that of pentobarbital. Antiemetic effects are not a prominent action of the benzodiazepines.
2. On respiratory system: It causes a dose related central respiratory system depression. This is greater with imidazole. The peak onset of ventilatory depression with midazolam is rapid and significant depression remains for about 60–120 minutes. This is more so in patients with chronic obstructive pulmonary disease. Occasionally apnoea occurs with benzodiazepines. Apnoea is more related to the dose of benzodiazepines and more likely to occur in presence of opioids.
3. On cardiovascular system: The predominant haemodynamic changes is a slight reduction in arterial blood pressure, resulting from a decrease in systemic vascular resistance. Baroreflex is impaired with both midzolam and diazepam. Midazolan causes slightly more decrease in blood pressure than other benzodiazepines. Heart rate, ventricular filling pressures and cardiac output are maintained after induction of anaesthesia with benzodiazepines. The stresses of endotracheal intubation and surgery are not blocked by midazolam. They decrease catecholamines.

Uses

(A) Intravenous sedation: They are used for sedation as preoperative premedication, intraoperatively during regional or local anaesthesia and postoperatively. The drugs should be given by titration for this use; end points of titration are adequate sedation or dysarthria. The onset of action is more rapid with midazolam. Lorazepam is particularly unpredictable with regard to duration of amnesia and this is undesirable in patients who wish or need to have recall in the immediate postoperative period. Prolonged infusion will result in accumulation of drug and in case of midazolam, significant concentration of active metabolites.

(B) Induction and maintenance of anaesthesia: Midazolam is of choice for use in anaesthetic induction. Advantages are faster onset of action and lack of venous complications. With midazolam, induction of anaesthesia is defined as unresponsiveness to command and loss of eyelash reflex. Factors affecting the dose are speed of injection, degree of premedication, age, ASA status and concurrent anaesthetic drugs. When midazolam is used with other anaesthetic agents, there is a synergistic interaction and the induction dose is less than 0.1 mg/kg. The synergy is seen when midazolam is used with opioids and/or other hypnotics such as thiopental and propofol. This complication therapy is called conduction. Awakening after benzodiazepine anaesthesia is the result of redistribution of drug from brain to other less well perfused tissues. The emergence defined as orientation to time and place in young patients who received 10 mg intravenous midazolam occurs in about 15 minutes. Benzodiazepines lack analgesic properties and must be used with other anaesthestic drugs to provide sufficient analgesic. The amnesic period after an anaesthetic dose is about 1 to 2 hours.

Side Effects and Contraindications

They have high margins of safety, especially compared with barbiturates. They are free from all allergenic effects and don't suppress adrenal gland. Most significant problem with midazolam is respiratory depression. Major side effect and lorazepam and diazepam are venous irritation and thrombo phlebitis, problems related to aqueous insolubility and requisite solvents.

PROPOFOL
Introduction

Propofol is the most recent intravenous anaesthetic to be marketed from clinical use. The favourable pharmacokinetic profile makes it suitable for both induction andextension, by repeated bolus or infusion to the maintenance of anaesthesia with easy and responsive titration to effect and rapid recovery.

Pharmaceutics

It's an alkylphenol, 2-6-disopropylphenol. It's highly soluble in lipid but not water and is formulated as an aqueous emulsion with intralipid, specifically an isoqueous emulsion with intralipid, specifically an isotonic 1% solution with 10% soyabeen oil, 2.25% glycerol and 1.2% purified egg phosphatide. This is stable at room temperature and not light sensitive. The addition of disodium edetate 0.005% suppresses bacterial growth without compromising the clinically safety, efficiacy and stability. The drug license specifies acceptable combinations and conditions of use.

Pharmacokinetics

The initial volume of distribution is 20–40L and distribution half-life 1–8 min. Following an intravenous bolus, plasma levels initially decline rapidly, due to redistribution of propofol from highly perfused, low capacity tissues, including the brain, to high capacity tissues with lower perfusion. Subsequent metabolic clearance is extremely large. The large volume of distribution at a steady state results in a long elimination half-life estimated to be in between 4 to 23.5 hours. Clinical recovery from propofol sedation or anaesthesia that has been titrated to therapeutic effect is relatively fast. It is rapidly metabolised by liver by conjugation to produce inactive, water-soluble glucuronide and sulphate compounds which are excreted by kidneys. The hepatic extraction ratio is high: Propofol degradation is more dependent on liver blood flow than on metabolism.

Pharmacodynamics

A commercial system for the target controlled infusion of propofol has been marketed i.e., Diprifusor 24. This delivers a predicted plasma propofol concentration and not the desired drug effect. The operating anaesthesiologist must estimate the target plasma concentration required to achieve the desired effect. This depends upon the extent of surgical stimulation.

Actions

1. On central nervous System: Propofol causes dose dependent sedation and hyposis. Amnesia is poor compared with barbiturates. Propofol is associated with an elevation of mood and a general state of well being 25. Hallucinations and sexual fantasies are reported. The EEG effects include a transient b excitation at low doses followed by a concentration dependent decrease in median. EEG frequency and an increase in EEG amplitude leading to burst suppression at high blood concentrations. The excitatory effects include occasional involuntary movements, myoclonus, dystonic posturing and opisthotonos. They are subscortical in origin and not associated with epileptiform EEG activity. It has dose-dependent anticonvulsant properties, reduces the motor and EEG seizure activity during ECT. It is sensibly avoided in patients with history of seizures for whom an unexpected grand mal seizure would be very dangerous. It reduces $CMRO_2$ and cerebral blood flow. Also causes decreased intracranial pressure in patients with normal or elevated ICP 26.

2. On cardiovascular system: It causes significant and concentration dependent decrease in arterial blood pressure during induction of anaesthesia. A fall in cardiac output is caused by myocardial depression and reduced ventricular filling pressures of a decrease in

systemic vascular smooth muscle tone. The relative fall in systemic blood pressure is not a big problem in healthy patients. It can be minimized by adequate preoperative hydration.

3. On respiratory system: It causes respiratory depression with a rise in arterial carbon dioxide tension and a reduced ventilatory response to both carbon dioxide and hypoxia. Apnoea is more common following an induction dose.

4. Other effects: Pain of injection into small peripheral veins occurs in many patients although not associated with phlebitis. This can be distressing and radiates proximally above the elbow. It causes a greater degree of relaxation of laryngeal muscles and better conditions for airway instrumentation.

Advantages
- Pleasant sedation and recovery.
- Rapid onset and easy titration effect.
- Suitable for both induction and maintainer of anaesthesia.
- Suppression of airway reflexes.
- Antiemetic effect and safe in porphyria.

Disadvantages
- Pain on injection.
- Lipid emulsion carrier, which supports bacterial growth.
- Vasodilation causes hypotension.
- Expensive.

Ketamine

Introduction

It is the only clinically useful phencyclidine derivative marketed for clinical use. This group of drugs is characterised by an unusual "dissociative" anaesthetic state profound analgesia, cardio respiratory stability and troublesome psychomimetic effects during recovery.

Pharmaceutics

It is presented as a racemic mixture of two optically active isomers, S (+) and R (–), in equal amounts. It is a clear colourless soluiton containing 1%, 5% or 10% ketamine hydrochloride with a pH of 3.5 to 5.5 These aqueous solutions are not irritating and ketamine can be administered by the intramuscular, extradural and intrathecal routes.

Pharmacokinetics

Low molecular weight, low protein binding a pKa close to the physiologic pH and high lipid solubility all contribute to very rapid penetration of the blood-brain barrier and onset of effect. The duration of anaesthesia following a typical intravenous anaesthetic dose of 24 mg/kg in an adult is 10–15 min, with recovery to full orientation in 1–30 min. The dependence of recovery time on the dose and duration of infusion is relatively small and similar to that of propofol and etomidate. It can be administered intravenously, intramuscularly, orally and rectally. Following intramuscular administration, onset of sedation occurs within 5 minutes and peak effect within about 20 minutes. Topical anaesthetic creams and modern volatile agents have reduced the trauma of induction of anaesthesia for children and their parents. The principal metabolite of N-demethylation by hepatic microsomal enzymes is nor ketamine. It is pharmacologically active but with less than of the potency of ketamine. Diazepam competitively inhibits N-demethylation of ketamine, decreasing its hepatic clearance.

Pharmacodynamics

1. On central nervous system: It produces an unusual cataleptic state with profound analgesia called 'dissociative anaesthesia,. The end point of induction being unclear; eyes

may remain open and corneal, gag and swallowing reflexes are well preserved. Non-competitive antagonism of glutamate at N-methyl-D-aspartate (NMDA) ligand gated calcium channels accounts for most of the anaesthetics analgesic, amnestic and psychotomimetic effects [27]. Inhibition of neuronal voltage gated sodium channels provides a modest local anaesthestic effects. It produces increased cerebral metabolism, cerebral oxygen consumption and cerebral blood flow. The consequent rise in intracranial pressure is particularly marked in the presence of intracranial pathology and hence it's contraindicated in patients with raised intracranial pressure and with intracranial pathology with a mass effect. There is parallel increase in intraocular pressure which may be detrimental in patients with open eye injuries or glaucoma or during vitreoretinal surgery. Emergence reactions include vivid dreams, surreal experiences and illusions with excitement and exophoria or unpleasant confusion and fear. The incidence is higher in adults than in children, in woman compared with men and in patients with a previous history of psychological problems. The patient start froms the same thought which he had before induction.

2. **On cardiovascular system:** Ketamine stimulates the cardiovascular system, with increases in heart rate, arterial pressure and cardiac output. The mechanisms is a centrally mediated increase in sympathetic tone and circulating catecholamines. The propensity for tachycardia and hypertension means it should be carefully used in patient with ischaemic heart disease or vascular aneurysms.

3. **On respiratory system:** It produces minimal respiratory depression and an unaltered response to carbon dioxide at clinically useful concentrations. Functional residual capacity, minute volume, tidal volume and the coordi-nated contribution of intercostal muscle function to inspiration are maintained. It has a clinically useful bronchodilating effect and has been useful in life threatening and unresponsive status asthmatics. Increased salivary and trachea bronchial secretions can be troublesome particularly in children. They may promote laryngospasm on airway obstruction but can be minimized by antisialayogues i.e., glycopyrrolate.

4. **Other effects:** Anaesthetic dose of ketamine increase uterine tone and the intensity of uterine contraction. Sympathetic stimulation and maintenance of cardio–vascular tone makes it a potentially life saving anaesthetic for parturients with exsanguinating obstetric haemorrhage and a flaccid uterus. It has been safely used for patients with malignant hyperthermia and acute intermittent and variegate porphyria.

Advantages
- Dissociate anaesthesia and marked analgesia.
- Very rapid onset of effect.
- Cardio respiratory stability.
- Relative preservation of airway reflexes.
- Safe in patients with porphyria.

Disadvantages
- Unpleasant and troublesome psychomimetic emergence reactions, lead to drug abuse in USA (Slow K). So it is banned in USA.
- Tachycardia and hypertension.
- Contraindicated by raised intracranial pressure.
- Heavy sedation and tongue falls postoperatively, leads to hypoxia. So should be avoided inchildren and patients of day care surgery and places where postoperative care is not adequate.

ETOMIDATE

Introduction

It is a potent, short acting intravenous anaesthetic, characterised by haemodynamic stability, minimal respiratory depression and cerebral protective effects.

Pharmaceutics and Physicochemical Properties

It is an imidazole derivative. Although presented as a racemic mixture, only the (+) isomer is an active hypnotic. It's insoluble in water and formulated in 35% propylene glycol as a 2 mg/mL solution. This mixture has low pH i.e., 5.6 and high osmolality. This is responsible for the frequent occurrence of pain on injection (30%) and superficial thrombophlebitis (20%) particularly when injected into small peripheral veins. Haemoglobinuria is undesirable with pre-existing renal disease. The total dose must not exceed 30 mL. Reformulation in lipofundin, a lipid emulsion (Etomidate lipuro) has solved much of its problems.

Pharmacokinetics

It rapidly crosses the blood brain barrier, producing peak effect site concentration within 1 minute of administration and a similarly fast onset of hypnosis. Moderate initial and steady state volumes of distribution and high redistribution clearance and metabolic clearance, both contribute exceptionally to short halflives of redistribution and elimination. This pharmacokinetic profile is ideally suited for rapid recovery.

Metabolism

Its rapidly metabolism in the liver primarily by ester hydrolysis, to the carboxylic acid derivative, which is inactive. The extraction ratio is high and metabolic clearance is hence dependent on liver flow.

Pharmacodynamics

It has hypnotic but not analgesic activity. The main sites of action appears to lie within the neocortex and its primary effects involve inhibition of the GABAergic system [28].

1. **On central nervous system:** A high incidence of myoclonus (50–80% is seen during induction of anaesthesia with etomidate in absence of premedication. Although usually self-limiting and of short duration, it can persist beyond recovery of consciousness. This is the subcortical effect, associated with slow and wave EEG activity indicating deep anaesthesia and no epileptiform EEG activity. Myoclonus can be reduced with pretreatment with low dose of etomidate, opioids or benzodiazepines. It shows potent anticonvulsants properties. It lowers cerebral blood flow (36%) and oxygen consumption in cerebrum (45%). Intracranial and intraocular pressure are substantially reduced. Cerebrovascular reactivity is maintained and hyperventilation further reduces intracranial pressure. Free haemoglobin produced by haemolysis secondary to propylene glycol may be scavenging local vasodilating nitric oxide.
2. **On cardiovascular system:** It minimally affects haemodynamic stability and myocardial function in healthy patients. Even in patients with moderate cardiac dysfunction, etomidate produces only minor cardiovascular changes, typically less than 10% decrease in cardiac index. Control of the sympathetic and haemodynamic response to laryngoscopy requires large doses of etomidate and synergistic doses of intravenous opiate.
3. **On respiratory system:** It has few ventilatory depressant properties than propofol and thiopental. Apnoea occurs less frequently. Hiccups and coughing are noted.

4. **Endocrine effects:** It causes suppression of adrenal cortisol synthesis. It is a dose-dependent but reversible inhibitor of 11 b-hydroxylase in the adrenal cortex. This enzyme is required for both mineralocorticoid and corticosteroid production. The effect of single bolus is short lived i.e., 6–8 hours.

Adverse Effects

Nausea and vomiting are common for etomidate with an incidence of 30–40%. This has severely limited the use of etomidate for day case surgery and it should be avoided in patients with increased risk of postoperative nausea-vomiting. It inhibits aminolevulinic acid synthetase and hence administered to patients with porphyria without precipitating a clinical crisis.

Advantages
- Haemodynamic stability.
- Reduction of $CMRO_2$, CBF and ICP with maintenance of CPP.
- Very rapid onset of hypnosis and recovery.

Disadvantages
- Hyperosmolar propylene glycol carriers cause pain on injection.
- Thrombophlebitis and haemolysis.
- Profound but transient inhibition of steroid oogenesis.
- Excitatory effects and myoclonus common.
- Postoperative nausea and vomiting.

New Intravenous Anesthetic drugs: Molecular biological research has made enormous progress in the identification, sequencing and cloning of ligand-gated ion channels in the central nervous system [29].

New Uses for Established Classes of Drugs

Derivatives of 5 and 5 reduced progesterone have anaesthetic properties. These drugs are characterised by a short duration of action and have a high therapeutic ratio for cardio respiratory depression. Eltanolone, also called prenanolone was formulated as an emulsion in Intralipid. A low incidence of nausea and vomiting, good cardiovascular stability and minimal respiratory depression were attractive features. However, involuntary movement and hypertonus, slow effect site equilibration and onset of action and a higher than expected incidence of urticaria were problematic and hence was discontinued [30]. Two water soluble, experimental imidazobenzodizepines i.e., RO 48-6791 and RO 48-8684 have been evaluated. Compared with midazolan, both drugs showed a higher clearance, a larger volume of distribution and a faster effect site equilibration [31].

Racemic Intravenous Anaesthetics

Enantiomers may share similar chemical properties but the specificity of their interactions with the clinical centres of receptors and enzymes produces pharma-cokinetic and pharmacodynamic differences. S-ketamine (+) is a more potent anaesthetic and analgesic and produces fewer psychosomatic emergence reactions than racemic ketamine. R-ketamine (−) acts as a competitive partial agonist at the effector site and competitively inhibits the metabolism of S-ketamine (+). Separation of pure enantiomers from a racemic mixture is an expensive manufacturing process and S-ketamine (+) is not commercially viable at present.

Reformulation of etomidate in a lipid emulsion reduced the incidence of pain on haemolysis were evident. Potency, pharmacokinetic profile and the inhibition of adrenal steroidogenesis were unchanged. The develop-ment of new intravenous anaesthetics is limited by enormous cost of development, manufacturing difficulties, protracted animal and human studies.

The prospects of improving the ways in which existing drugs are used are more promising. Synergism between drugs can be quantified and applied in clinical practice for benefits of patients [32]. The commercial target controlled infusion of propofol i.e., diprifusor uses a pharmacokinetic model to achieve a selected plasma concentration. Computer controlled infusion systems which incorporate mathematical models of effect site, kinetics are widely used in research.

REFERENCES

1. Van Dyke RA, Chenoweth MB, and Van Poznak A. Metabolism of volatile anaesthetics. I Conversion in vivo of several anaesthetics to 14CO-2 and Chloride. Biochem Pharmacol 1964; 13:1239.
2. Merkel G, and Eger EI (II). A comparative study of halothane and halopropane anaesthesia-including a method for determining equipotency. Anesthesiology 1963; 24:346.
3. Priestly J. Experiments and observations on different kinds of air London 1974.
4. British oxygen Ltd Co. Current methods of commercial production of nitrous oxide. Brit J Anaesth 1967;39:440.
5. Bourne, JG (1954). General anaesthesia for outpatients with special reference to dental extraction. Proc. Cory Se. Med 1954; 47:416.
6. Bloch M. Some systemic effects of nitrous oxide. Brit J. Anaesth 1963; 35:631.
7. Hassen HCA, Henriksen E. Neukrich F. and Kristen Sen HS. Treatment of tetanus. Severe bone marrow depression after prolonged nitrous oxide anaesthesia. Lancet 1956; 527.
8. Kumar P, Srivastava A. Ether Convulsion[5]. Asian Arch Anaesth Resus XIV 108;1982.
9. Barach AL and Rovenstine EA. The hazards of anoxia duirng nitrous oxide Anesthesiology 1945;6:449.
10. van Dyke RA, and Chenoweth MR. Metabolism of volatile anaesthetics II, Biochem. Pharmacol 1965; 14L603.
11. Ikezono E, Yasudo U and Hattori Effects of propanolol on epinephrine—Induced arrythmias during halothane anaesthesia in Man. Anesthe Analg. Curr. Res 1969;48:558.
12. Standford BJ, Plantevin OM and Gilbert JR. Morbidity after day case gynaecological surgery. Comparison of enflurane with halothane. Brit J Anaesth 1979; 51:1143.
13. Wolfson B. Hetric, WD Lake, CL and Siker ES. Anaesthetic indices. Further data. Anesthesiology 1978; 48:187.
14. Bentley JB, Vaughn RW, Miller M S Calkins JM and Gandolfi AJ. Serum inorganic fluoride levels in obese patients during and after enflurane anaesthesia Anesth Analg (Cleve) 1974; 58:409.
15. Stevens WC, Dolan WMb, Gibbons, RT, White A, Equer EI, Miller RD, De Jong RH and Elashoff RM. Minimum alveolar concentrations (MAC) of isoflurane with and without nitrous oxide in patients of varous ages. Anesthesiology. 1975; 42:197.
16. Nakajina R, Nakajina Y. Ikdeda K.Miniumm alveolar concentration of sevoflurane in elderly patients. Br J. Anaesth 1993; 70:273–5.
17. Holaday DA, Smith FR. Clinical charcteristics of biotransformation of sevoflurane in healthy human volunteers. Anesthesiology 1981; 54:100–6.
18. Rampill IJ, Lockhart SH, Zwass MS, et al. Clinical characteristics of desflurane in surgical pateints: Anesthesiology 1991; 74:429–33.
19. Healy TEJ, Cohen PJ, Wylie and Churchill-Davidson. A practice of anesthesia, 7th edn,. London, Arnold 2003.

20. Reddy RV, Moorthy SS, Dierdorf SF, et al. Excitatory effects and electroencephalographic correlation of etomidate, thiopental, methohexital and propofol. Anesth Analg 1993;77L1008–11.
21. Cheng MA, Theard MA, Temperhoff R. Intravenous agents and intra operative neuroprotection. Beyond barbiturates. Crit Care Clinic 1997; 13:185–99.
22. Brown GW, Patel N, Ellis FR. Comparison of propofol and thiopentone for LMA insertion. Anaesthesia 1991;46:771–2.
23. Baird ES, Hailey DM. Delayed recovery from a sedative: Correlation of the plasma levels of diazepam with clinical effects of oral and intravenous administration. Br J. Anaesth 1972; 44:803–8.
24. Mohler H, Richards JG. The Benzodiazepine receptor a pharmacological control element of brian function. Eur J Anaesthesiol (Suppl) 1988; 2:15–24.
25. Shafer SL. Advances in propofol pharmacokinetcs and pharmacodynamis. J Clin Anesth 1993; 5 (suppl).: 145–215.
26. Glass PS. Prevention of awareness during total intravenous anaesthesia. Anesthesiology 1993; 78:399–400.
27. Herregods L, Verbeke J, Rolly G, Colardyn F. Effects of propofol on elevated intracranial pressure. Preliminary results. Anaesthesia 1988; 43 (Suppl): 107–9.
28. Kohrs R, Durienx ME. Ketamine: Teaching an old drug new tricsk. Anesth Analg 1998; 87:1186–93.
29. Ostwarld P. Doencike A> Etomidate revisited. Curr Opin Anaesthesiol 1998; 11:391–8.
30. Lees G. Molecular mechanisms of anaesthesia: light at the end of the channel Br J. Anaesth 1998; 81:491–2.
31. Sear JW. Eltanolone: 50 years on a still looking for steroid hypnotic agents: (Editorial) Eur J Anaesthesiol 1998; 15:129–32.
32. Dingemanse J, Hanssler J, Herinjf W, et al. Pharmacokinetic Pharmacodynamic modelling on the EEG effects of R 48-6791, a new short acting benzodiazepine in young and elderly patients. Br J. Anaesth 1997; 79:567–74.
33. Vinki HR. Intravenous anaesthetic drug interactions: Practical applications. Eur J anaesthesiol 1995; 12 (suppl):13–9.
34. Kumar P. Drugs in anaesthesia. 1st Edn, New Delhi Modern Publishers, 2006.
35. Kumar Pramod. Anaesthesia for Dentistry. 1st Edn. New Delhi. Modern Publishers, 2006.
36. Kumar Pramod Anaesthesia for veternay and reasearch animals. 2st Edn, New DelhiCBS Publishers, 2006.

Chapter 6. Local Anaesthetics

Local anaesthetics produce transient loss of sensory, motor and autonomic function in a discrete portion of body.

Local Anaesthetic Action

Nerve cells maintain a resting membrane potential by active transport and passive diffusion of ions. The sodium potassium pump transports sodium out of the cell and potassium into the cell. This creates a concentration gradient that favours extracellular diffusion of potassium and intracellular diffusion of sodium. The cell membrane is much more permeable to potassium than to sodium, however, a relative excess of negatively charged ions (anions) accumulate intracellularly. This accounts for the negative resting potential difference (–70 mV polarization). After chemical, mechanical or electrical excitation, an impulse is conducted along a nerve axon. The impulse propagation is usually accompanied by depolarization of nerve membrane. If the depolarization exceeds the threshold level (i.e. –55 mV), sodium channels in the membrane are activated allowing a sudden and spontaneous influx of sodium ions. This increase in sodium permeability causes a relative excess of positively charged ions (cations) intracelluularly, resulting in membrane potential of +35 mV, a consequent drop in sodium permeability (created by inactivation of sodium channels) and an increase in potassium conductance (allowing more potassium to exit the cell) return the membrane to its resting potential. Baseline concentration gradients are eventually re-established by sodium potassium pump. These changes in axon membrane potential are collectively called the action potential. Most local anaesthetic bind to sodium channels in the inactivated state preventing subsequent channel activation and the large transient sodium influx associated with membrane depolarization. This does not alter the resting membrane potential or the threshold level, but it slows the rate of depolarization. The action potential is not propagated because the threshold level is never attained. Specific receptors in the interior of the sodium channels are probably the exact site of local anaesthetic action (Fig. 1).

Some local anaesthetic may penetrate the membrane, causing membrane expansion and channel distortion.

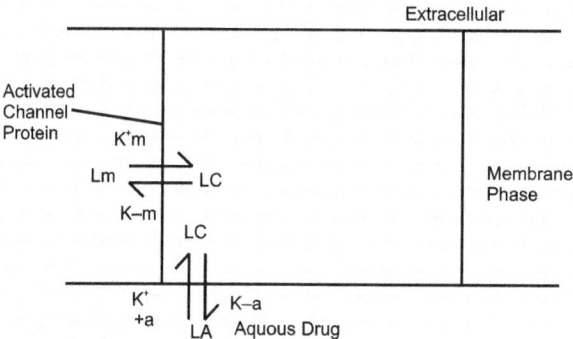

Fig. 1: Drug access routes to a L.A. binding site on Na^+ channel

Alternately the surface charge theory postulates that partial penetration by local anaesthetics of the axonal membrane could increase transmembrane potential and inhibit depolarization.

Structure Activity Relationships

Local anaesthetics consists of a lipophilic group (usually a benzen ring) separated from a hydrophilic group (usually a tertiary amine) by an intermediate chain that includes an ester or amide linkage (Fig. 2). Local anaesthetics are weak base that usually carry a positive charge at the tertiary amine group at physiological pH. The nature of the intermediate chain is the basis of the classification of local anaesthetics as either esters or amides. Physicochemical (Tables 1 and 2) properties of local anaesthetics depend on substitution in the aromatic ring, the type of linkage in the intermediate chain and the alkyl groups attached to the amine nitrogen.

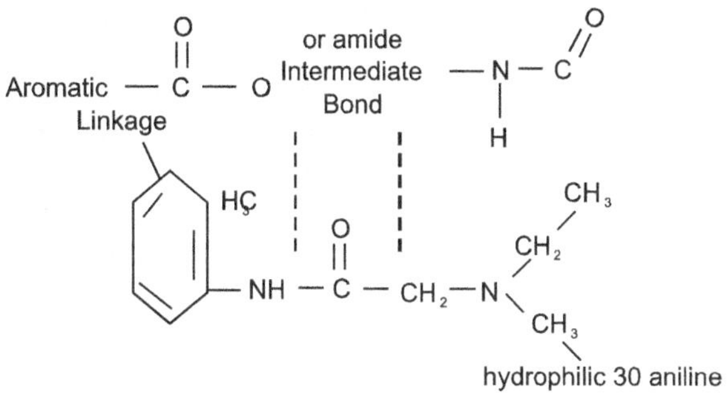

Fig. 2: Local anaesthetic Molecule

Potency correlates lipid solubility, that is, potency depends on the ability of the local anaesthetic to penetrate the hydrophobic environment, potency and hydro-phobicity increases with increase in the total number of carbon atoms in the molecule. More specifically, potency is increased by adding a halide to the aromatic ring (2-chlorprocaine as opposed to procaine), an ester linkage (procaine versus procainamide) and large alkyl groups on the tertiary amide nitrogen (etidocaine versus lignocaine). (Fig. 3 alveolar concentration (MAC) of inhalational anaesthetics, (Cm is the minimum concentration of local anaesthetic that will block nerve impulses conduction. This measure of relative potency is affected by several factors, including fibre size, fibre type and myelination, pH (acidic pH antagonizes block); frequency of nerve stimulation (access of local anaesthetic to sodium receptor is enhanced by repeatedly opening the sodium channel); and electrolyte concentrations (hyperkalaemia and hypercalcaemia antagonize block).

Onset of action depends on many factors, including relative concentration of the nonionized lipid form (B) and ionized, water soluble form (BH^+). The pH at which the amount of ionized and nonionized drug is equal to the pK^a of the drug.

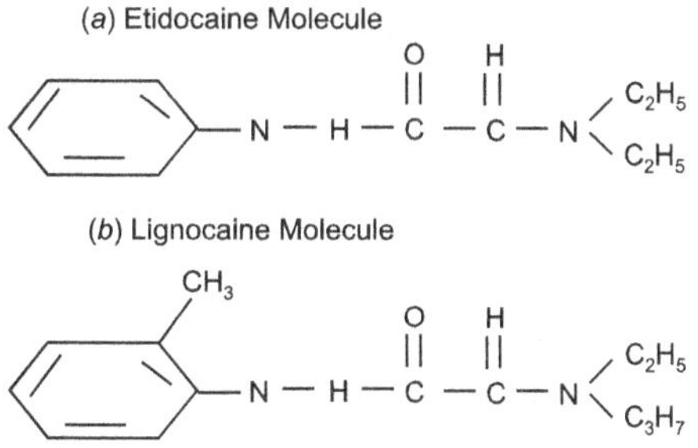

Fig. 3 : (a) Etidocaine and (b) ligocaine molecule

Although both forms of local anaesthetic are involved in blockade, only the lipid soluble form diffuses across the neural sheath (epineurium)) and nerve membrane. Local anaesthetics with a pK^a closer to physiologic pH will have a higher concentration of non- ionized base that can pass through the nerve cell membrane and the onset will be more rapid. Once inside the cell, the

Table 1 : Comparative pharmacology of local anaesthetics

Classification	Potency	Onset	Duration (mins)	Maximum dose mg	Toxic plasma (*mg/mL)	pK_a
Esters						
Procaine	1	Slow	45–60	500		8.9
Chloroprocaine	4	Rapid	30–45	600		8.7
Tetracaine	16	Slow	60–180	100 (topical)		8.5
Amides						
Lignocaine	1	Rapid	60–120	300	>5	7.9
Etidocaine	4	Slow	240–480	300	~2	7.7
Prilocaine	1	Slow	60–120	400	>5	7.9
Mepivacaine	1	Slow	90–180	300	>5	7.6
Bupivacaine	4	Slow	240–480	175	~1.5	8.1
Ropivacaine	4	Slow	240–480	200	~4	8.1

Table.2: Use of local anaesthetics to produce regional anaesthesia

Elimination	Fraction nonionized (%)			Protein binding	Lipid solubility	Volume distribution (liters)	Clearance (liters/min)	half-time (mins)
	pH 7.2	pH 7.4	pH 7.6					
Esters								
Procaine	2	3	5	6	0.6			
Chloro-procaine	3	5	7					
Tetracaine	5	7	11	76	80			
Amides								
Lignocaine	17	25	33	70	2.9	91	0.95	96
Etidocaine	24	33	44	94	141	133	1.22	156
Prilocaine	17	24	33	55	0.9			
Mepivacaine	28	39	50	77	1	84	9.78	114
Bupivacaine	11	15	24	95	28	73	0.47	210
Ropivacaine	8.1			94		41	0.44	108

Table 3: Routes of local anaesthetics to produce regional anaesthesia

	Topical anaesthesia	Local infiltration	Peripheral nerve block	Intravenous regional	Epidural anaesthesia	Spinal anaesthesia
Procaine	No	Yes	Yes	No	No	Yes
Chloroprocaine	No	Yes	Yes	No	Yes	No
Tetracaine	Yes	No	No	No	No	Yes
Lidocaine	Yes	Yes	Yes	Yes	Yes	Yes (?)
Etidocaine	No	Yes	Yes	No	Yes	No
Prilocaine	No	Yes	Yes	Yes	Yes	No
Mepivacaine	No	Yes	Yes	No	Yes	No
Bupivacaine	No	Yes	Yes	No	Yes	Yes
Ropivacaine	No	Yes	Yes	No	Yes	Yes
Pramaxine	Yes	No	No	No	No	No
Dyclonine	Yes	No	No	No	No	No
Hexylcaine	Yes	No	No	No	No	No
Piperocaine	Yes	No	No	No	No	No

nonionized base will reach in equilibrium with the ionized form. Only the charged cations actually bind to the receptor within the sodium channel.

The importance of the ionized and nonionized form has many clinical implications. Local anaesthetic solutions are prepared commercially as water-soluble hydrochloride salt (pH 6–7). Because adrenaline is unstable in alkaline environments, local anaesthetic solutions containing it are made even more acidic (pH 4-5),. Because of lower concentration of free base these have slower onset of action than when adrenaline is used. The extracellular base-to-cation ratio is decreased and onset is delayed when local anesthetics are injected into acidic (infected) tissus.

Tachyphylaxis is explained by the eventual consumption of local extracellular buffering capacity by the acidic local anaesthetic. Conversely, if carbonated solutions of local anaesthetic rather than the hydrochloride salts are used, onset of action may be shortened. This appears to be due to improved intercellular distribution of ionized form. Although controversial, alkalinization of anaesthetic solution (particularly commercially prepared solutions containing adrenaline epinephrine that tend to be acidic) by addition of sodium bicarbonate (e.g., 1 Mole (M) 8.4% sodium bicarbonate per 10 mL of 1% lignocaine) speedy onset, improves quality of block and prolongs it. The combination also decreases pain during subcutaneous infiltration.

Onset of action of local anaesthetics in isolated nerve fibre preparations directly correlates with pK_a.

Duration of action is associated with plasma protein binding (acid glycoprotein) presumably because the local anaesthetic receptor is also protein. The pharmacokinetics also affects duration of action.

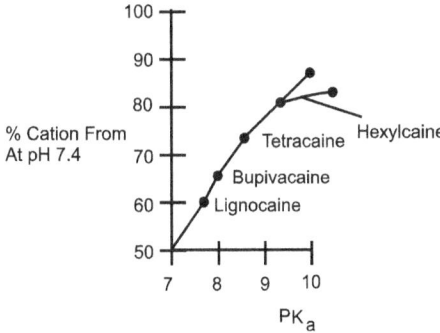

Fig. 4: Cationic form and pK_a of LA

Liposomal encapsulation systems for delivery of local anaesthetics may significantly prolong duration of action.

Bupivacaine in lower concentrations produces less motor block due to effect on less susceptible senssory efferents sparing C fibres (Fig. 4).

Clinical Pharmacology

Pharmacokinetics

A. Absorption

Traditionally, local anaesthetics have been applied to mucous membrane (e.g., ocular conjunctiva) or injected into a variety of tissues and compartments. Most mucous membranes provide a weak barrier to their penetration, leading to rapid onset of action. Skin although requires a high water concentration for its penetration and a high concentration of lipid soluble local anaesthetic base to ensure analgesia. EMLA cream (euletic mixture of local anaesthetic) consists of 1% mixture of 5% lignocaine and 5% prilocaine in oil and water emulsion. Dermal analgesia sufficient for beginning an intravenous line requires a contact time of at least 1 hour under occlusive dressing. Depth of penetration 3–5 mm), duration of action (usually 1–2 hours), and amount of dry absorbed depends on application time, dermal blood flow, keratin thickness and total dose administration. 1-2 g of cream is applied per 10 cm^2 area of skin with a maximum application area of 2000 cm^2 in an adult (100 cm^2 for children less than 10 kg). Split thickness skin graft harvesting laser removal of postcrine strains, lithotripsy and circumsicion have been successfully performed with EMLA cream. Side effects include skin branching, erythema and oedema with cream not to be used on mucous membranes, broken skin, infants less than 1 month old or patients predisposed to methaemoglobinaemia. Table .4 shows concentrations used.

Systemic absorption of injected local anaesthetic depends on blood flow, which is determined by the following factors:

Table 4: Local analgesic actions

Drug	Concentration %	Infiltration Max dose	Duration	Conc%	Nerve blocks Max. Dose	Duration
Chloroprocaine	1.2	800	15.30		100	30
Lignocaine	0.5–1	300	30–60		200	60–120
Bupivacaine	0.25–0.5	175	120–240		50–100	180–360
Etidocaine	0.5–1.0	300	120–180		100–200	120–260

1. Site of injection: The rate of systemic absorption in proportionate to the vascularity of site of injection: intravenous > tracheal > intercoastal > caudal > paracervical > epidural > branchial plexus > sciatic > subcutaneous.
2. Pressure of vasoconstrictiors: The addition of vasoconstrictiors like epinephrine causes vasocon-striction at the site of administration leading to decreased absorption, increases neuronal uptake, enhancing the quality of analgesia, prolonging duration of action and limiting toxic side effects. The effect of vasoconstrictors is more pronounced with shorter acting agents like lignocaine.
3. Local anaesthetic agents

Local anaesthetics that are highly tissue bound are more slowly absorbed (e.g., etidocaine). The agents also vary in their intrinsic vasodilator properties.

B. Distribution

Distribution depends on organ uptake, which is determined by following factors:
1. Tissue perfusions: Highly perfused organs like brain, lung, heart etc., are responsible for initial rapid uptake (alpha phase), which is followed by slower redistribution (beta phase) to moderately perfused tissues (muscle and gut). The lung in particular, extract significant amount of local anaesthetics.
2. Tissue/blood partition coefficient:
   Strong plasma protein binding tends to retain anaesthetic in the blood, while high lipid solubility facilitates tissue uptake.
3. Tissue mass: Muscle provides the greatest reservoir for local anaesthetic agents because of large mass.

C. Metabolism and Excretion

The metabolism and excretion on of local anaesthetic differs depending on their structure.
1. Ester: Esters are predominantly metabolized by pseudocholinesterase (plasma cholinesterase). Ester hydrolysis is rapid and the water soluble metabolites are excreted in urine. One metabolite, P-aminobenzoic acid, has been associated with allergic reactions. Patients with genetically abnormal pseudocholinesterase are at increased risk of toxic side effects, since metabolism is slower. Cerebrospinal fluid lacks esterase enzyme, so the termination of action of intrathecally administered local anaesthetic depends on their absorption into the blood stream. In contrast, cocaine is partially metabolized in liver and partially excreted unchanged in urine.
2. Amides: Amides are metabolized by microsomal enzymes in liver. The rate of metabolism depends on specific agent (prilocaine faster than lignocaine, which is faster than bupivacaine) but is much slower than ester hydrolysis. Decrease in the hepatic function as in cirrhosis or

liver blood flow as in CHF will reduce metabolic rate and predispose patients to systemic toxicity. Very little drug is excreted unchanged in urine, although the metabolities are depend on renal clearance. Metabolities of prilocaine (co-toluidine derivatines) which accumalate after large doses of drug (> 10 mg/kg), convert haemoglobin to methaemoglobin. Neonates of mother who receive the drug in epidural anaesthesia during labour and patients with limited cardio-pulmonary reserves are particularly susceptible to alteration in oxygen transport. Treatment includes intravenous administration of methylene blue (1-2 mg/kg of 1% solution over 5 minutes), it reduces methaemoglobin (Fe^{3+}) to haemoglobin (Fe^{2+}).

Effects on Organ System

Local anaesthetics have the capacity for systemic toxicity. Toxicity is often directly proportional to dose, potency and mixture of LA should be considered to have roughly additive toxic effects.

A. Cardiovascular

In general, local anaesthetics depress myocardial automaticity (spontaneous phase IV depolarization) and reduce the duration of refractory period. Myocardial contractility and conduction velocity are depressed at higher concentrations (Fig. 5). These effects results from direct cardiac muscle membrane changes (i.e., cardiac sodium channel blockade) and inhibition of autonomic nervous system. Smooth muscle relaxation causes some degree of arteriolar dilatation. The ensuing combination of bradycardia, heart block and hypotension may simulate cardiac arrest. Cardiac dysrhythmia or circulatory collapse is often the presenting sign of local anaesthetic overdose during general anaesthesia (Table .5). Lower concentration of lignocaine provides effective treatment of some types of ventricular dysrhythmia. Myocardial contractility and arterial blood pressure are generally unaffected by usual intravenous doses. The hypertension associated with laryngoscopy and intubation is attenuated in some patients by intravenous administration of lignocaine (1.5 mg/kg) 1–3 minutes prior to instrumentation.

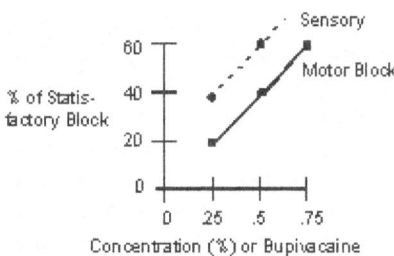

Fig 19.5: Differential sensory and Motor blockade

Table 5: Effect of LA or cardiac output

Drug	Relative Potency	Cardiac output (mg/Kg (50%))
Procaine	1	100
Lignocaine	2	30
Bupivacaine	8	10
Etidocaine	6	25

Unintentional intravascular injection of bupivacaine during regional anaesthesia has produced severe cardiotoxic reactions including, hypotension, arterio-ventricular heart block and dysrythmias such as ventricular fibrillation. Pregnancy, hypoxaemia and respiratory acidosis are predisposing risk factors. Bupivacaine is associated with more pronounced depolarization changes than lignocaine. Bupivacaine blocks cardiac sodium channels and alters mitochondrial function. Its high degree of protein binding makes resuscitation prolonged and difficult.

Ropivacaine a relatively new amide local anaesthetic, shares many physiochemical properties with bupi-vacaine except that it is half as lipid soluble. Potency, onset time and duration of action are similar. However, ropivacaine has a larger therapeutic index because it is 70% less likely to cause severe cardiac dysrythmias than bupivacaine and ropivacaine has been assosiated with greater central nervous system tolerance. This improved safety profile may be due to its lower lipid solubility or its availability as a pure S (–) isomer, as opposed to bupivacaines racemic mixture. The S (–) isomer of bupivacaine (levobupivacaine) has been reported to have fewer cardiovascular and cerebral side effects than the racemic mixture. Otherwise, levobupivacaine and bupivacaine appear to exhibit similar anaesthetic effects. Cocaine inhibits nore pinephrine resorption by adrenergic nerve terminals thereby potentiating the effects of adrenergic stimulation. Cardiovascular responses to cocaine include hypertension and ventricular ectopy. The latter contraindicates its use in patients anaesthesised with halothane. Cocaine induced dysrythmias have been successfully treated with adrenergic and calcium channel antagonists. Cocaine produces vasoconstriction when applied topically.

B. Respiratory

Lignocaine depresses hypoxic drive. Apnoea can result from phrenic and intercoastal nerve paralysis or depression of the medullary respiratory centre following direct exposure to local anaesthetic agent. Local anaesthetics relax bronchial smooth muscle. Intravenous lignocaine (1.5 mg/kg) may be effective in blocking the reflex bronchoconstriction sometimes associated with intubation. Lignocaine administered as aerosol can lead to bronchospasm in some patients with reactive airway disease.

C. Neurological

The central nervous system is espacially vulnerable to local anaesthetic toxicity and is the site of premonitory signs of overdose in awake patients. Early symptoms are circumoral numbness, tongue paraesthesia and dizziness. Sensory complaints may include tinnitus and blurred vision. Excitatory signs (e.g., restlessness agitation, nervousness, paranoia) often precede central nervous system depression (e.g., slurred speech, drowsiness, and unconsciousness), muscle twitching heralds the onset of tonicoclonic seizures. Respiratory arrest often follows. The excitatory reactions are a results of selective blockade of inhibitory pathways. By decreasing cerebral blood flow and drug exposure, benzodiazepines and hyper ventilation raise the threshold of local anaesthetic induced seizures. Thiopental (1–2 mg/kg) quickly and reliably terminates seizure activity. Adequate ventilation and oxygenation must be maintained.

Intravenous lignocaine (1.5 mg/kg) decreases cerebral blood flow and attenuates the rise in intracranial pressure that accompanies intubation in patients with decreased intracranial compliance. Infusion of lignocaine and procaine has been used to supplement general anaesthetic techniques, since they are capable of reducing the MAC of volatile anaesthetics by upto 40% (Fig. 6).

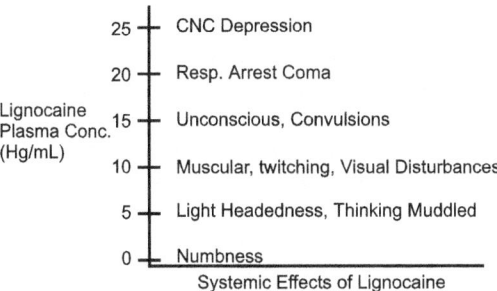

Fig. 6: CNS side effects of Lignocaine concentration

Cocaine stimulates the central nervous system and usually causes a sense of euphoria. An overdose is heralded by restlessness, emesis, tremors, convulsions and respiratory failure. Local anaesthetics only temporarily block neuronal function.

Repeated doses of 0.5% lignocaine and 0.5% tetracaine may be responsible for neurotoxicity (cauda equina syndrome) following infusion through small bore catheters used in continuous spinal anaesthesia. This may be due to pooling of drug around the cauda equina, resulting in high concentrations and permanent neuronal damage.

Transient neurologic symptoms, which consists of dysaesthesia, burning, pain and aching in the lower extremities and buttocks' have been reported following spinal anaesthesia with a variety of local anaesthetics. The aetiology of symptoms has been associated to radicular irritation and symptoms typically resolve within a week.

Risk factors include lignocaine, lithotomy position, obesity and outpatient status.

D. Immunologic

True hypersensitivity reactions to local anaesthetics as distinct from systemic toxicity caused by excessive plasma concentration are quite uncommon. Esters are more likely to induced allergic reactions because they are derivatives of p-aminobenzoic acid, a known allergen. Commercial multidose preperations (amide prepara-tions) contain methylparaben which has a chemical structure similar to that of p-aminobenzoic acid, is responsible for most of the rare allergic reactions to amides. Local anaesthetics may inhibit neutrophil function and theoretically retract wound healing.

E. Musculoskeletal

When directly injected into skeletal muscle local anaesthetics are myotoxic (bupivacaine > lignocaine > procaine). Histologically, myofibril hyper contraction progress to lytic degeneration oedema and necrosis. Regeneration usually occurs after 3–4 weeks. Concomitant steroid or epinephrine injection worsens myonephrosis.

F. Haematologic

Lignocaine has been demonstrated to decrease coagulation (prevention of thrombosis and decrease platelet aggregation) and enhance fibrinolysis of whole blood as measured by thromboelastography. These effects may relate to the reduced efficacy of epidural autologous blood patch shortly following local anaesthetic administration and the lower incidence of embolic events in patients receiving epidural anaesthetics.

Drug Interactions

1. Nondepolarizing muscle relaxant blockade is potentiated by local anaesthetics.

2. Succinylcholine and ester local anaesthetics depend on pseudocholinesterase for metabolism. Concurrent administration may potentiate the effect of both drugs.
3. Dibucaine an amide local anaesthetic, inhibits pseudocholinesterase and is used to detect genetically abnormal enzymes.
4. Pseudocholinesterase inhibitors can lead to decreased metabolism of ester local anaesthetics.
5. Cimetidine and propanol decrease hepatic blood flow and lignocaine clearance. Higher lignocaine blood levels increase the potential for systemic toxicity.
6. Opioids (e.g., fentanyl, morphine) a_2–adrenergic agonists (e.g., epinephrine clonidine) potentiate local anaesthetic pain relief. Epidural chloro-procaine may interfere with analgesic action of intraspinal morphine, however, as may bupivacaine with fentanyl.
7. Cocaine is the only L/A which consistently causes vasoconstriction at all concentration due to its ability to inhibit the uptake of norepinephrine by storage granules and thus potentiate neurogenic vasoconstriction.
8. Some studies have found increases in pulmonary vascular resistance from local anaesthetic infusion.

Lignocaine hydrochloride (BP.) (Xylocaine, Lidocaine)

Diethylamino-2: 6-dimethylacetanilide, is the commonly used drug. A basic anilide, synthesized by Lotgren and Lundquist (Astro) in 1943 in Sweeden. First used by Gordh in 1948. It is very stable, not decomposed by boiling, acids or alkalies. Its onset is quicker and duration is longer than that of procaine. It seems to spread over a wider field than equal volumes of other analgesics. Solutions of 0.25 to 0.5% for infiltration, with adrenaline 1–250,000 4% for topical analgesia in ENT. For nerve block 1.5 to 2% with adrenaline and for extradural block 1.2 to 2% with adrenaline. For corneal analgesia 4% without causing mydriasis, vasoconstrction or cycloplegia. For urethral analgesia 1 to 2% in jelly and for endotracheal tubes 2% jelly.

Metabolism of lignocaine can give rise to the formation of methaemoglobin, The average peak concentration ensuing within 4–6 hours after 0.8% injection. Cynosis is very rare. It is not a vasodilator nor interferes with vasoconstrietion of adrenaline. Cerebral effects can be drowsiness and amnesia. It is metabolised by microsomes in the liver, chief metabolite being diethylaminoacetic acid which is excreted renally.

Lignocaine interacts with phenytoin leading to sinoatrial arrest of the heart. Duration one hour with 1% solution, 1½ hours with adrenaline.

It has been used I.V. to treat ventricular arrythmia by membrane stabilising action. Also used in status epilepticus. However, it is less successful in multiple ectopic foci.

Maximum safe dose–3 mg/ kg body weight (200 mg) and 7 mg per kg when used with adrenaline. A solution of 20–40 mL can be used in 0.5–1%.

Bupivacaine (Sensorcaine): Synthasized by E.K. Stam in 1957 and used clinically by Telivuo in 1963. The hydrochloride is dissolved in water. It was developed from mepivacaine, the methyl group in the pipericline ring being replaced by a butyl group. It is four times as potent as mepivacaine and lignocaine (0.5% solution is equal to 2% Lignocaine). It causes sensory, more efficiently than motor block. The margin of safety with supivacaine appears to be wider than above drugs when used extradural. Duration of action is between 2–3½ hours by spinal route which is due to binding to lipoprotiens of nerve tissue than to its overall retention in the body. A small percentage of this drug is excreted unchanged in the urine. The N-dealkylated metabolite pipecolyloxylidine, is found in the urine. The maximal dose is 2 mg/kg b.wt (25–30 mL of 0.5% solution) a 0.25–0.5% The adrenaline does not prolong its effect. The pH of 0.5% solution is 3.5 with a density of 0.997 g / mL at 37°C.

Uses: For prolonged extradural block, brachial plexus, digtital block, caudal and intercostal block in concentration of 0.5%, 10 to 30 mL.

Sodium Channel and Local Anaesthetics

Most of the available local anaesthetics act by blocking the nerve impulse propagation by stabilizing the sodium channel. The present local anaesthetic drugs are safe, effective and convenient but for their potentially useful or unwanted effects. The exploration of local anaesthetics of cocaine family may not be fruitful but the present knowlege of structure of target sodium channel may permit the construction of a tailor made antagonist molecule that would precisely target the channel. Antibody with their huge molecules can be effective antagonist. So the effort is on to skillfully identify that part of the large molecule which is active in achieving specificity of control. This opens up possibility of newer channel blockers which are shaped to affect nerve membrane alone and thus will be more specific.

Some naturally occurring sodium channel blockers are:
1. Tetradotoxin (TTX) found in puffer fish and vents.
2. Sexitoxin found in denoflagellate and insect clams.
3. Maculotoxin comes from saliva of Australian octopus.

Tetrodotoxin (TTX) : It is 1,00,000 times more potent than cocaine. It blocks inputs at so low concentration that there are not sufficient TTX moles to go around for each sodium channel. This means that there are single receptors present in the nerve membrane which in turn influence stability of other sodium channel. TTX is a small, complex molecule which is difficult to synthesize.

Other effects: There are some effects other than overdose toxicity due to blockade of motor and autonomic fibres. Arner et a wrote a paper on prolonged relief of neuralgia after regional anaesthetic blocks.
Thirty–eight patients after peripheral nerve injury received 5–10 mL of 0.5% bupivacaine. There was 12 hour analgesia in 26 patients, 15 hour in 18 patients and 2–6 days analgesia in 5 patients. This study went unnoticed by and large by the scientific community, but explained the neuralgic pain relief out of proportion to the sensory motor effects and the doses used.

Immediate effect of blocking sensory nerve impulses: Dental phantom, phantom limb: It is explained on a nerve cell as follows. There is a steady tonic input from periphery which is in part inhibitory normally. When that input is blocked, central cells expand their receptive fields and immediately begin to respond to novel inputs and increase their excitability. There is a compensatory increase of excitability perhaps by a degree of inhibition, leading to deafferentation. This is more marked in unmyelinated C fibres. This is not to be confused with the phantom limb.

Local anaesthetic effects
A. **Nerve block effects:** Immediate: 1. Blockade of transmission of nerve impulses. 2. Phantom phenomenon in the area of the blocked nerve. 3. Expansion of receptive field by central neurons leading to increased neuronal excitability by decreased inhibition, normally activated by tonic inputs from C fibres. 4. Effects of local anaesthetics at the site of the application or via systemic absorption: The effects are anti-inflammatory, decrease ectopic impulses in the damaged nerve, reduce ectopic impulses in the dorsal root ganglion, reduced slow and rapid axonal transport systems, decrease noradrenaline reuptake in spinal cord with analgesic effect at spinal cord level, cardiac membrane stabilization in muscles and nerves and CNS effects of hyperalgesia in low concentration and convulsions at high concentrations.

B. Pre-emptive effects: A volley of impulses in spinal cord in unmyelinated fibres triggers response in dorsal horn, leading to excitability due to release of amino acids and peptides. These in turn excite cells and trigger a cascade of changes in cell membrane and nucleus, e.g., entry of calcium ions, unmasking of NMDA–receptors, release of nitric oxide and novel proteins. These changes last for many hours and marked with excitability and can be prevented by nerve blocks. For example, post- operative pain is due to central barrage of impulses produced by surgery during operation and can be blocked by pre-emptive analgesia. This pre-emptive effect is clear in animals has to be investigated further in humans.

C. Chronic effects: In these conditions impulse blockade is present for days, weeks and months. The presence of pattern impulse in the input in case of both eyes (convergent), which is accurately timed to produce binocular overlap. This is disturbed in squint and rearing in dark. The other example is disuse of atrophy of muscle. It is not certain if a similar phenomenon exists in sensory system. Apart from impulse generation the transport system is also effected. Another example is tenotomy, which presents silent proprioceptive input in shortened muscle resulting in radical change of entire reflex circuit supplying the affected muscle. These changes in impulse patterns or transport are not very well known in adults. In normal case, hippocampus is related to learning and memory.

Inflammation

The anti–inflammatory action of local anaesthetics have been currenlty studied extensively. The action is thought to be by the blockade of nerve impulses which trigger release of substance P into the surrounding tissue. The substance P leads to vasodilation, swelling and sensitization of nerve endings by separate processes and secondly by blocking impulses in sympathetic axons. This also influences mobility of white cells from the surrounding tissues and blood leading to infiltration.

Damaged neurons

The damaged nerve becomes: 1. Sensitive to α– adrenergic action (an action more in myelinated nerves) leading to ectopic impulses. This action is blocked by subclinical blocking doses. 2. Prolongation of refractory period of excitation for impulse generation of high frequency, while sparing low frequency impulses *e.g.,* touch. After damage, the dorsal horn receives abnormal inputs from the area of damage and from DRG cells (which also send ectopic impulses after damage). The DRG cells react to α– adrenergic action and are more sensitive to local anaesthetics than the damage area.

Transport in nerve fibres

Transport in the nerve fibres is by slow and fast transport systems, which need energy to move protein and peptide molecules, which in damaged nerve accumulate on proximal site of damaged axon. The distal part of the axon develops Wallerian degeneration.

Some Newer Local Anaesthetics

Levobupivacaine

Bupivacaine is a racemic mixture of two enantiomers (R) (+) and S (–) most commonly used epidurally. There is stereospecificity of action of CNS or CVS. So S (–) enantiometer levobupivacaine was developed, which is better tolerated. Racemic bupivacaine produces greater prolongation of QRS complex, vasoconstriction, detrimental in vascular beds (decreases uterine blood flow) an action not seen with levobupivacaine.

It increases the duration of sensory block, variable spread of subarachnoid and epidural (1.5 mL of 0.5%) blockade.

No difference in quality of surgical anaesthesia, no ventilatory depression. In labour, analgesia more patients require second injection earlier.

Sameridine

Isobaric greater time to reach peak height, failure rate higher, with duration of block shorter than lignocaine.

Less preoperative analgesia needed (4 hours, lower VAS score). Similar time to void and ablate as lignocaine.

Onset slower than lignocaine. Side effects: ventilatory response to increase in CO_2 and VO_2 is less. No respiratory depression, mild pruritus, increased QTc interval.

Butyl Aminobenzoate

Its pK_a is low, is less water soluble with poor dural permeability and rapid hydrolysis. Prepared in polyethylene glycol or polysorbates. Selectivity of A delta and C fiber, minimal motor block with sparing of bladder and bower functions. Low lipid solubility, increased duration of action and there is a slow release.

Liposome (L)

Encapsulated local anaesthetic and opioid analgesic preparations. Prolongs duration of action of bupivacaine and morphine.

Duration of action: 2–3 times more than bupivacaine.

Anatomy of Peripheral Nerve

Each peripheral nerve possess its own cell membrane.

Non-myelinated nerves such as autonomic postganglionic and nociceptive afferent fibres are encased in a single Schwann cell sheath (Fig. 7).

- Most large motor and sensory fibres are enclosed in many layers of myelin which consists of plasma membrane of specialized Schwann cells that wrap around the axon during axonal outgrowth. Myelin increases the speed of nerve conduction by insulating the axolemma from the surrounding conducting medium forcing the action current to flow through axoplasm to the node of Ranvier which are periodic interruptions[9] in the myelin sheath where the action currents are regenerated.

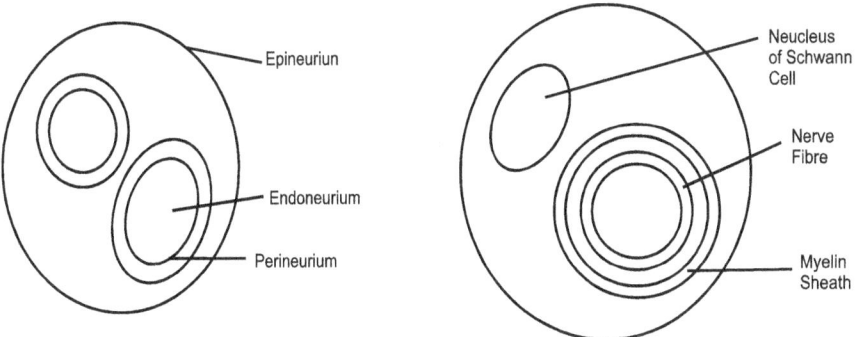

Fig. 7: (a) Transverse section of a peripheral nerve (b) Myelinated axons

Structure of Axonal Membrane (Figs. 8)

Biologic membrane consists of a molecular lipid bilayer containing protein on the structure as well as embedded in or sparing the hydrocarbon core. The bilayer character is imposed by the aminophilic phospholipids, which have long hydrophobic fatty acid sites that lie in the centre of membrane and polar hydrophilic head group composed of component that projects into the cytoplasm or the interstitial blood.

Physiology of Nerve Conduction

The neuronal membrane is found to monitor a voltage difference of 60–90 mV between its inner and outer aspects because at rest it is relatively impermeable to Na^+ ions but is selectively permeable to K^+ ion.

An active energy dependent mechanism the Na^+ K^+ pump sustains the gradients that maintains this potential difference by constant exchange of Na^+ from the cell in exchange for a net uptake of K^+ using ATP as an energy source.

The nerve at rest behaves as a K electrode according to the equation.

$$Em = \text{Membrane potential}$$
$$EK = \text{Potassium equilibrium potential}$$
$$R = \text{Gas Constant}$$
$$T = \text{Temperature (kelvin)}$$
$$F = \text{Faraday's constant}$$
$$EK = -58 \log 30$$
$$\text{or} = 85.7 \text{ mV}$$

An opposite situation exists for Na^+ which is at higher concentration outside the cell and has a nearest potential $E\,Na^+$ 60 mV.

During an action potential the membrane transiently switches its permeability from K^+ selective to Na^+ selective thus changing the membrane potential from –ve to +ve and back again.

Sodium channels, in addition, close to an inactivated conformation following their initial activation.

A small membrane depolarization exists along an axon from a region of excited membrane for e.g., beginning to open both Na^+ and K^+ channels.

The Na^+ channels open faster, however, because the membrane potential is initially much farther from the nearest potential for Na^+ than for that of K^+. Inwardly directed Na^+ current is larger.

Na^+ is entering the nerve and depolarizes it further leading to opening of more Na^+ channel and increases the current further.

The sequence of events continues in the +ve feedback of the depolarizing phase until some of Na^+ channels have become inactivated and enough of K^+ channel have opened to change the balance of arrest, resulting in a net outward current but produces membrane repolarization (Fig. 8).

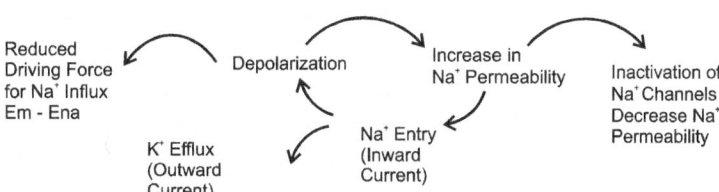

Fig. 8: Factors contributing to regeneration of depolarisation of action potential

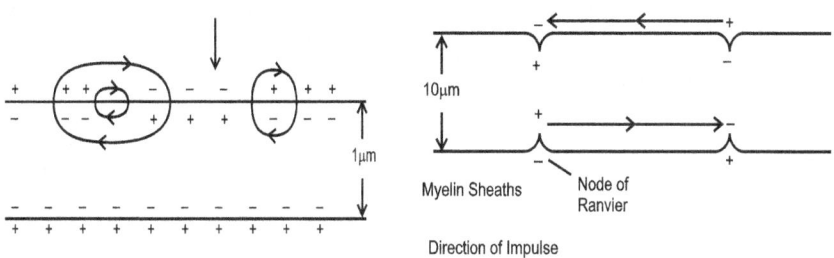

Fig. 9: Action current flowing in (a) Nonmyelinated nerve (b) Action current flowing in myolinatd nerve

In the immediately repolarized membrane as Na^+ inactivation decays, K^+ channels return to their closed conformation, the original value is progressively reached. (Fig. 8 shows factors contributing to regeneration of depolarization.)

The impulse is a wave of depolarization that is propagated along the axon by a continuous coupling between excited and non-excited parts of membrane.

Ionic current (action current) entering the axon in the excited depolarized region flow down the axoplasm and exits through the surrounding membrane thus passively depolarizes the adjacent region.

Although this local current spreads, away from the excited zone in both directions, the region behind the impulse has just been depolarized and is in absolute refractory state and impulse propagation is thus uni- directional.

The local circuit currents spread rapidly along a length of insulated intermediate area in a myelinated axon and nodes of Ranvier in sequence or depolarized to threshold level with little intervening delay. Fig. 9 shows action current flowing in (a) non myelinated or (b) myelinated nerves.

Single impulse don't jump from node to node as separate discrete event, but instead the active depolarization occurs simultaneously along axon. Indeed the local circuit current is so that it can skip two completely non-excited nodes and may successfully stimulate a nerve.

If node excitability is partially reduced by inhibition of some of the Na^+ channels for exchange, the amplitude of impulses in successive nodes follow decrementation of a process than can continue for cm.

This situation probably occurs during certain phases of LA. block.

The inhibition of Na^+ channels is sufficient so that local circuit current fails to bring the adjacent resting regions to threshold, then the impulse is extinguished.

Prolonged Infusions of Local Anesthetics, Tachyphylaxis and Development of Long Duration Local Anesthetics

Local anaesthetics are increasingly being administered by continuous infusion for several days after surgery or for periods of weeks to months for the treatment of chronic malignant and nonmalignant pain. With proloned infusions, there is potential for delayed systemic accumulation and toxicity. Continuous infusions of bupivacaine of up to 30 mg/hr in adults for up to 2 weeks produced no overt CNS or cardiac toxicity despite total plasma bupivacaine concentrations in the range of 2 to 5 mg/mL in several patients.

Apparent reductions in the effectiveness of local anaesthetic infusions may be due to a number of causes unrelated to tolerance per se, including dislodgement of epidural catheters and changes in the dermatomal origin or intensity of nociceptive input. In obsetetric patients receiving epidural bolus injections, recurrence of pain before the next injection resulted in a reduction in the intensity and duraion of blokade, wheras repeat injection before the return of pain prevented this rapidly occurring form of tolerance, or tachyphylaxis. In post-operative patients, the coadministration of systemic opioids prevented regression of segmental blockade in patients receiving thoracic epidural bupivacaine infusions. Studies in rats suggest that both pharmacokinetic and pharmacodynamic mechanisms are involved. In a rat model, tachyphylaxis was linked to the development of hyperalgesia and drugs that inhibited hyperalgesia, including N-methyl-D-aspartate receptor antagonists and nitric oxide synthase inhibitors, 216 also prevented tachyphylaxis. Conversely, repeated sciatic injections of lidocaine produced reduced intraneural lignocaine content along with a reduced duration of block.

Several methods are under investigation to produce long-duration nerve blockade. Liposomal encapsulation, as mentioned, can prolong blockade, depending on the dose and the physical properties of the liposome (surface charge, size, lamellar structure). Local anaesthetics can be incorporated into biodegradable polymer micro-spheres for sustained release. These preparations produce peripheral nerve block in animal models ranging from 2 to 8 days, depending on the dose, site, and species.

Prolonged-duration local anaesthesia also appears to be feasible with the use of site 1 sodium channel toxins in combination with either local anaesthetics or adrenergics. Other drugs have been examined for use as local anaesthetics, including tricyclic antidepressants. It remains to be determined whether local anaesthetics with prolonged duration will receive widespread use in clinical practice. If they prove safe and effective, they may have potential use in intercostal blockade and wound infiltration, particularly for surgery. If drugs can be developed that last for weeks or longer, they may have additional applications in the management of chronic pain and cancer pain.

Clinical Tips- Local anaesthetics block voltage-gated sodium channels by interrupting the initiation and propagation of impulses in axons, but they have a wide variety of other biologic actions, both desirable and undesirable.

The currently available local anaesthetics are of two chemical clases: aminoesters and aminoamides.

The low potency and lack of specificity of the available local anaesthetics are due in part to the structural constraint that they must have high solubility and diffuse rapidly in both aqueous environments and the lipid phases of biologic membranes.

Reversible protonation of the tertiary amine group makes local anaesthetics uncharged at basic pH and charged at acid pH; the base forms are more soluble in lipid environments, whereas the acid forms are more soluble in aqueous environments.

Aminoesters are primarily metabolized by plasma esterases; aminoamides are metabolized primarily by hepatic cytochrome P450-linked enzymes.

The principal systemic toxicities of local anaesthetics involve the heart (including atrioventricular conduction block, arrhythmias, myocardial depression and cardiac arrest) and the brain (including irritability, lethargy, seizures, and generalized CNS depression). Hypoxaemia and acidosis exacerbate these toxicities. Resuscitation after bupivacaine overdose is particularly difficult. Therefore, prevention of intravascular injection or overdose is crucial, and major nerve blockade should involve incremental, fractionated dosing.

Local anaesthetics are directly toxic to nerve at the concentrations supplied in commercial solutions.

Intraneural concentrations during regional anaesthesia are generally (but not always) below the threshold for toxicity because of spread of solutions through tissues and diffusion gradients from injection sites into nerve. Injection into a constrained tissue space increases the risk of local toxicity.

Optimal use of local anaesthetics in regional anaesthesia requires an understanding of the individual patient's clinical situation the location, intensity, and duration of regional anaesthesia and alnagesia required; anatomic factors affecting the deposition of drug near nerves; proper drug selection and dosing; and ongoing assessment of clinical effects after administration of local anaesthetics.

REFERENCES

1. Strichartz G. Handbook of experimental pharmacology. Local anesthetics. Heidelberg, Springer, 1987.
2. Miller RD. Anesthesia. 5th Ed, Philadelphia, Churchill Livingstone, 2003.
3. Covino B. Pharmacology of Local anaesthetic agents Br. J Anaesth 1986;58:701.
4. Prys Roberts C, Hug CJ. Pharmacokinetics of Anesthetics, Oxford, Blocknell scientific Publications. 1984.
5. Covino B, Vesselato H. Local anaesthetics. Mechanism of Action and Clinical use. Orlando, Fla, Grune and Stratton, 1976.
6. Kumar P. 6 Recent advances in regional anaesthesa and analgesia Asian Arch Anaesth. Resus 2005, LXIII, (2) 1251-1258.
7. Kumar Pramod. A Text book of Pain. 1st Edn, New Delhi, Modern Publishers, 2005.
8. Kumar Pramod. Drugs in Anaesthesia. 1st Edn, New Delhi, Modern Publishers, 2006.

Chapter 7   NON STEROIDAL ANTI INFLAMMATORY DRUGS (NSAIDS)

For more than 100 years little was known abut the mode of action of NSAIDS are the predominant group of drugs, used to reduce pain and inflammation. This group has been enlarged recently by the introduction of selective cyclooxygenase – 2 these compounds. Within last 50 years a coherent pharmacological picture has been created. The discovery of prostaglandins synthesis does not explain as to why aspirin and (acidic) NSAIDs exert anti-inflammatory and analgesic effects while non-acidic pyhenazone and acetaminophen are analgesic only[1]. All acidic anti-inflammatory are highly bound to plasma proteins with pK_a between 3.5-5.5. A high protein binding and an open endothelial layer of vasculature there is a high concentration in the inflamed tissue, GIT, Kidney and block the COX-2 locally. By contrast neutral pK_a value drugs like phenazone are evenly distributed throughout the body. These acidic NSAIDs cause acute side effects in GIT (ulcer) blood stream (inhibition of platelet aggregation) kidney (fluid and K^+ retention) and respiratory mucosa (asthma) {fig. 1}

Table 1: Acidic NSAIDs (Brune and Lanz, 1985)[3]

Sub class	pKa (protein binding)	Time to peak plasma concentration	Elimination half life	Single dose range (max. daily dose)
Low potency ➤ Aspirin ➤ Salicylic acid ➤ Ibuprofen	3.5 2.9 4.4	-0.25h 0.5-2h 0.5-2h	20min 2.5-7h 2-4h	0.05-0.1g(6g) 0.5-1g(6g) 0.15-100g(300g)
High potency ➤ Acetyl proprionic acids (ketoprofen, blurbiprofen) ➤ Arylacetic acids (diclofenac) ➤ Indomethacin, ketorolac ➤ oxicams	4.2 4 4.5 4.9	0.5-2h 0.5-24h 0.5-2h 0.5-2h	1.1-4h 1-2h 2.6-11.2h 4-10h	15-100mg(300mg) 25-75mg(200mg) 25-75mg(200mg) 4-12mg (16mg)
Intermediate potency ➤ Salicylates diflunisal ➤ Arylproprionic acid ➤ Arylacetic acids 6MNA	3.8 4.15 2.4	2-3h 2-4h 3-6h	8-12h 13-15h 20-24h	250-500mg(1g) 0.5-1g(2g) 0.5-1g(1.5g)
High potency (slow elimination) ➤ Oxicams ➤ Tenoxicam	5.1 5.0	3-5h 3-5h	14-160h 25-175h	20-40mg(initially 40mg) 20-40mg

CYCLOEXYGENASES:

In 1991 two different genes code for cyclooxygenases COX1 and COX 2 were discovered, cloned, sequenced and characterised[4]. These enzymes form a hydrophobic groove or channel opening through the membrane, the substrate (arachidonic acid) or an inhibitor inserts into this groove. The COX2 proteins displays a larger channel than COX1[5]

Physio-pathology of COX-1&2: the COX1 isoenzyme is present in most tissues and produces prostaglandins. The COX2 is an inducible isoenzyme, which acts in inflammatory cells (e.g. Macrophages an synoviocytes) after exposure to proinflammatory cytokines and is down regulated by glucocorticoids. In the kidney (macula densa) and other areas of the urogenital tract and in the CNS, COX2 is significantly present, over in the absence of inflammation. Induction of COX2 beyond baseline levels in the peripheral nervous system and spinal cord is prominent in connection with inflammatory painful reactions. Both these enzymes are blocked by NSAIDs.

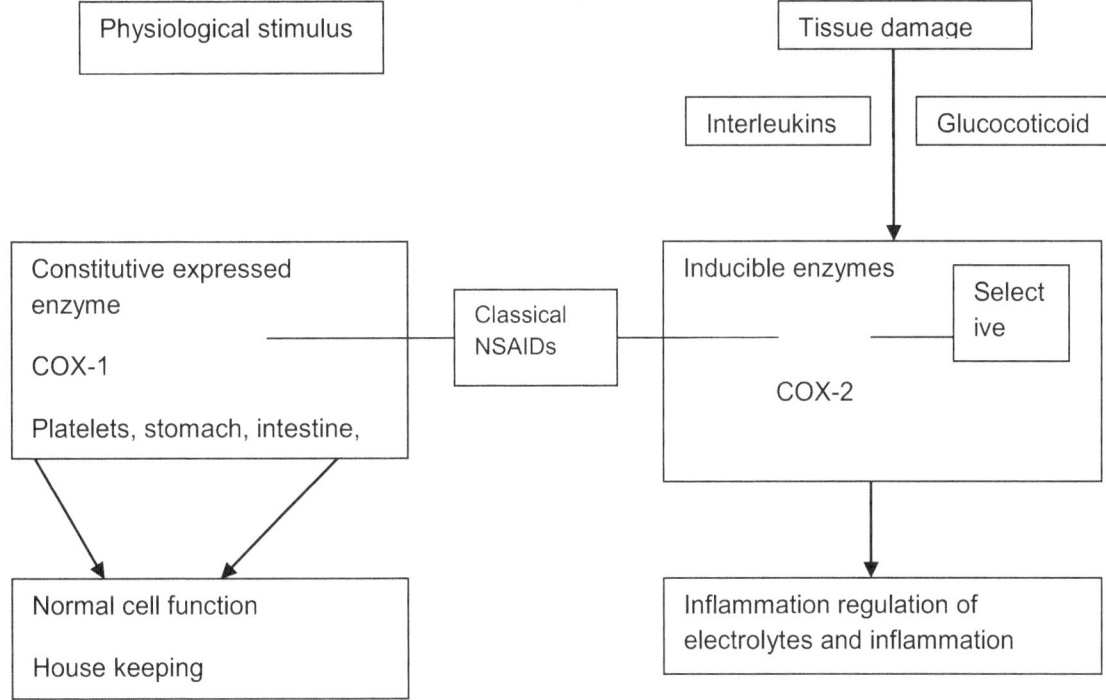

Fig 1: physio pathogenesis of COX-1 and COX-2 (Kay Bruce)[6]

Indications for NSAIDs

indications	High dose	Middle dose	Low dose
Acidic NSAIDs			
➢ Spondylitis, gout, arthritis	Diclofenac, indomethacin, piroxicam, ibuprofen	Diclofenac, indomethacin, piroxicam	No
➢ Cancer pain (bone)	Diclofenac, ibupro0fen, piroxicam, indomethacin	Diclofenac, ibuprofen, piroxicam, indomethacin	Acetyl salicylic acid, ibuprofen
➢ Active arthrosis			

(inflammation)	No		Ibuprofen, ketoprofen
➢ Myofascial pain	No	Diclofenac, ibuprofen, piroxicam, indomethacin	Ibuprofen, ketoprofen
➢ Trauma(swelling)	No	Diclofenac, ibuprofen, piroxicam, indomethacin	Ibuprofen, ketoprofen
➢ Post operative pain	No	Diclofenac, ibuprofen, piroxicam, indomethacin	Ibuprofen, ketoprofen
		Diclofenac, ibuprofen, piroxicam, indomethacin	
Non acid NSAIDs	Coxibs	Pyrozolinones	Anilines
➢ Acute pain and fever	?	Yes	No
➢ Spastic pain (colic)	?	Yes	No
➢ Associated with fever	?	Yes	Yes
➢ Cancer pain	yes	Yes	Yes
➢ Headache, migraine	?	yes	yes
➢ Associated viral infections			

Non acidic NSAIDs
Anilines

Most widely used drug of this drug of this group, acetaminophen (paracetamol) was discovered at the same time as aspirin. They are weak and possibly indirectly inhibitor of cycloexygenases. Specially at COX-2. 1g/kg/ b.w. doses it has few side effects except liver toxicity. Acetaminophen is metabolized to toxic nuecloephilic benzoquinones that bind to DNA and structural proteins in parenchymal cells in liver and kidney. Glutathione or N-acetyl cystine administration in early stages can prevent the liver necrosis. Indications are fever, mild pain in viral infections, recurrent headache and can be used in children.

Acetaminophen can be used in combination with aspirin and caffeine but can cause nephropathy.[8]

Phenazones (depyrone and propyphenazone)

Used as antipyretic and analgesics. They can lead to agranulocytosis. All antipyretics can cause Stevens- Johnson syndrome, Lyell's syndrome and shock reactions. All non acid NSAIDs are devoid of GIT and renal toxicity.

Table 3: NSAIDS

Pharmacological subdivision	Plasma protein binding	Time to peak concentration	Elimination half life	Single dose (daily dose)
Acetaminophen	5-50%	0.5-1.5hr	1.5-2.5hr	0.5-1g(1-6g)

paracetamol				
Phenazone (antipyrine)	<10%	0.5-2hr	5-24hr	0.5-2g(1-6g)
propylphenazone	10%	0.5-1.5hr	1-2.5hr	0.5-2g(1-6g)
Metamizole (depyrone)	20-50%	1-2hr	2-4hr	0.5-2g(1-6g)
Selective COX inhibitors Celecoxib Rofecoxib	>90% >80%	2-4hr 2-4hr	9-15hr 12hr	40-200mg(400mg) 12-25mg(25mg)

Prostaglandins and hyperalgesia:

The analgesic action of NSAIDs is due to inhibition of the production of prostaglandins at the site of inflammation and in the CNS. Prostaglandins sensitize primary afferent nerve C-fibers and there by activate the silent nociceptors causing primary hyperalgesia by targeting at the tetrodotoxin resistant Na+ channels. A peripheral inflammation stimulates prostaglandin in the dorsal horn of spinal cord leading to secondary hyperalgesia and allodynia[9]. the prostaglandin interferes with glycinergic inhibition in the spinal cord.

Inhibition of COX-2 activity by NSAIDs

The NSAIDs act at the COX active site which is at the end of a hydrophobic channel that runs from the membrane binding surface of the enzyme into the interior of the molecule.

- Aspirin irreversibly inactivates both COX-1&2 by acetylating an active site and thereby interfering with the binding of arachidonic acid in the active site
- However, ibuprofen compete with arachidonic acid for COX active site
- While flurbiprofen and indomethacin cause a slow, time-dependent, reversible inhibition of COX1&2 by formation of a salt bridge between carboxylate of the drug.

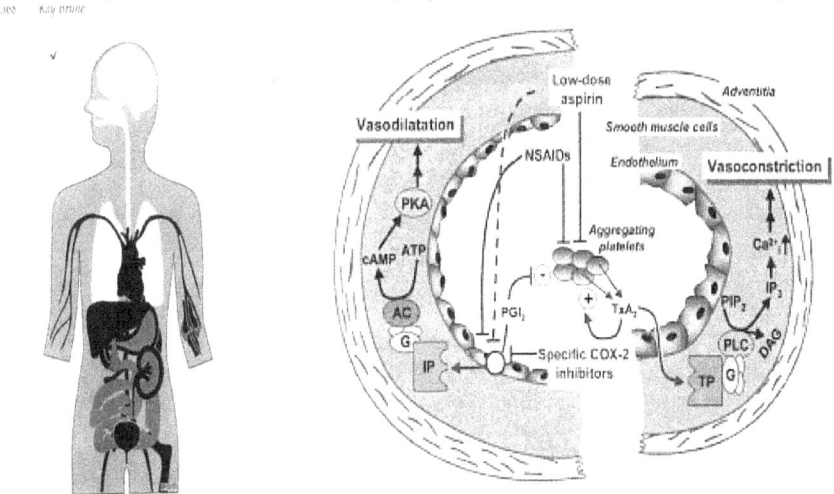

Fig 2 Distribution of acidic anti pyretic analgesics in the human body.(dark areas shows increased concentrations)

Fig.3. Regulation of peripheral vascular tone by prostacyclins and thromboxaneA2

Clinical use of acidic NSAIDs

Acidic NSAID compounds (aspirin) at high doses (>3g/day) inhibits not only pain and fever but also inflammation i.e. swelling redness and warming. These compounds differ in their potency, with single doses ranging between a few mgs (ornoxicam) to about 0.8 g (ibuprofen) and also differ in their pharmacokinetic characteristics (time to peak action and oral bioavailability). However these drugs lack a relevant degree of COX-2 selectivity (inhibitors of COX-2 at concentrations that does not block COX-1. That is why these drugs are classified according to their potency and elimination half life.

Selective COX-2 inhibitors: The slow absorption and elimination of Coxibs make them poor candidates for acute pain. However they are effective for osteoarthritis and rheumatoid arthritis. Both of them show analgesic potency comparable to that of traditional NSAIDs[9]

COX-2 and GIT:

Even in double clinical doses celecoxib and rofecoxib cause a significantly lower incidence of upper GIT due to the protective action of the prostaglandins secreted from COX-1. However there is some dyspepsia with an incidence lower than that seen with NSAIDs but higher than with placebo[10]. These drugs may influence ulcer healing buy interfering with associated angiogenesis.

COX-2 and kidney functions

COX-2 immunoreactivity was detected in renal vasculature, medullary interstitial cells and macula densa, whereas COX-1 was detected in the collecting ducts, loop of Henle and renal vasculature. This can offend renin-angiotensin system. Therefore COX-2 inhibitors can cause peripheral edema, hypertension and exacerbation of preexisting hypertension by inhibiting salt and water excretion by kidney. The prostacylin reduction can lead to reduced Na+ excretion comparable to other NSAIDs. So it is advisable to use them with caution in patients with fluid retention, hypertension and heart failure.

COX-2 and cardiovascular system

COX-2 inhibitors can alter the thromboxane-prostacyclin balance by inhibiting the vasoprotective prostacyclin in endothelial cells. This can lead to hyper coagulability. However these complications are comparable to other NSAIDs. However VIGOR study showed four fold increases in the incidence of myocardial infarctions as compared to naproxen[11] in patients with rheumatoid arthritis.So COX-2 inhibitors may provide a significantly improved risk benefit ratio in terms of GIT safety especially in old age patients and in patients receiving glucocorticoids and anticoagulants. However, available COX-2 inhibitors do not compare favorably with the old non acidic antipyretic analgesics e.g. Acetaminophen and propylphenazines.

References:

1. Graf. P, Glatt M, Brune K. Acidic nonsteroid anti-inflammatory drugs accumulating in inflammedtissue. Experientia, 1975, 31:951-954.
2. Day RO, Francis H, Vial J, Geisslinger G, Williams KM. Naproxen concentrations in plasma and synovial fluid and effects on prostanoid concentrations. J. Rheumatol.1995, 22:2295-2303.
3. Brune K, Lanz R. Pharmacokinetics of non-steroidal anti-inflammatory drugs. In: Bonta II, BrayMA, Parnham MJ(eds). The pharmacology of inflammation, handbook f inflammation, Vol. 5. Amsterdam: Elsevier, 1985, pp 413-449
4. O. Banion MK, Sadowki HB, Ninn V, Young DA. A serum and glucocorticoids regulated 4-kilohase m-RNA encodes a cyclo-oxygenase related protein. J. Biol. Chem 1991; 266 : 23261-23267
5. Kurumball RG, Steven Sam, Gierse JK. Structural basis for the selective inhibition of cyclooxygenase – 2 by anti-inflammatory agents. Nature 1996; 384:644-648.
6. Kaybrun E. Non opoid (antipyretic) analgesics. In; Pain 2002 an update review. Refresher course syllabus. Maria Adele, Ed. Giamberdiko, IASP press, Seattle, 2002m pp 365-379
7. Samad TA, Moore KA, Sapirstein A. Interleukin 1 beta-medicated inductin of COX-2 in the CNS contributes to inflammatory pain hypersensitivity. Nature 2001; 410: 471-475
8. Porter GA. Acetaminophen/ aspirin mixtures : experimental data Am. J. Kidney dis. 1996; 28(supp): 30-33
9. Fitzgerald GA, Patroro C. The coxibs selective inhibitors of cyclooxygenases 2. N. Engl. J. Med 2001: 345-34

Chapter 8. Opioids

The word opium is derived from the Greek word, juice of the poppy, from which twenty distinct alkaloids are formed.

The term narcotic is derived from the Greek word 'stuper' and generally refers to morphine like analgesics with the potential to cause physical dependence.

Opioids refer to all exogenous substances, natural or synthetic that bind to opioid receptors and produce atleast some agonist effects.

Structure

The opioid alkaloids are of two types (i) Phenanethrene (morphine, codeine, thebaine (ii) soquinalones (papavarine, noscapine).

The three rings of phenanthrene nucleus are composed of 14 carbon atoms. The fourth ring is piperidine ring, which includes a tertiary amine nitrogen, which at pH 7.4, is highly ionised, making the molecule, water soluble.

Semisynthetic opioids are result of semipre- modification of the morphine molecule, e.g., codeine, heroin, fentanyl, sufentanyl, alfentanyl, remifentanil, Synthetic opioid contain the phenanethrene nucleus of morphine, but are manufactured by synthesis e.g., fortwin, butorphanal.

Mechanism of Action

The opioids are agonists at stereo specific opioid receptor at presynaptic and postsynaptic sites in the CNS (brain stem and spinal cord) and in peripheral tissues e.g., primary afferent neurons.

Only the levorotatory forms of opioids show agonist activity.

Opioids act by causing increased potassium conductance, leading to hyper polarisation and also decrease in calcium release. Thereby, they cause presynaptic inhibition of neurotransmitters like acetylcholine, substance-P, dopamine and noradrenaline.

Opioid Receptors

They belong to a group of guanine (G) protein-coupled receptors[1] (Table 10).

They are classified as mu, delta, and kappa receptors.

Mu_1: Produce analgesia at supraspinal and spinal levels.

Euphoria, miosis, bradycardia, hypothermia, urinary retention.
Agonists- Endorphin, morphine, synthetic opioids.
Mu2: Spinal Analgesia, Respiratory depression, Nausea.
Agonists: endorphin, morphine, physical synthetic opioids depen-dance.

Kappa: Analgesia at spinal and supraspinal levels, dysphoria, sedation, diuresis, miosis.
Agonists: dynorphines. They have low abuse potential.

Delta receptors: They produce analgesia at spinal and supraspinal levels. Depression of ventilation, constipation, urinary retention. physical dependence
Agonists: Encephalin

SYSTEMIC EFFECTS

1. Cardiovascular System

The effects of opioids on any system is studied with morphine as the prototype.

Morphine, causes impairment of compensatory sympathetic nervous system response, and these causes venous pooling, thereby reducing the cardiac output and systemic blood presence.

Morphine, causes hypotension by stimulating the vagal nuclei in the medulla oblongata.

Table 3: Characteristics of opiate receptors[3].

	Mu	Delta	Kappa
Tissue bioassay	Guinea pig ileus	Mouse vas deferens	Rabbit vas deferens
Endogenous ligands	Encephalin endorphins (?)	Encephalin	Dynorphin
Exogenous agonist ligand	Morphine	DPDPE	50488
	phenylpiperidines	DADLE	Bremazocine
	Butorphanol		
	DAMGO, DAGO	Deltorphin	
Antagonist	Naloxone	Naloxone	Naloxone
	Naltrexone	Naltrindole	N or BNI
Cloned (human)	Yes	Yes	Yes
Subtypes	1,2,3	1,2,cx,ncx	1,2,1a,2a,b
G-protein coupled	yes	yes	yes
Adenylate cyclase[153]	Inhibits	Inhibits	Inhibits
Ca^{++} channels	Inactivates	Inactivate	Inactivates
K^+ channels conductance	Increases	Increases	Increases
Actions	Analgesia, sedation, respiratory depression, dysphoria, decreased nausea, vomiting and increased GI mobility	Supraspinal analgesia, miosis, bradycardia, Respiration	Diuresis, spinal analgesia, respiratory depression
Spinal cord	yes	yes	yes

It may also exert a direct effect on the sinoatrial node, these causing bradycardia and slow conduction through the atrioventricular node as well. This may, in part explain the decreased vulnerability to ventricula or fibrillation.

Opioid induced histamine release and associated hypotension are both variable in incidence and degree. This can be prevented by using smaller doses of the opioid (morphine < 5 mg/min IV) and optimising the intravascular fluid volume.

The opioid does not sensitize the heart to catecholamines, nor does it prevent the tachycardia and hypertension associated with painful surgical stimulation. However, it can be attenuated by using large doses of the opioid.

The combination of opioid agonists, such as morphine along with nitrous oxide or inhalational agents, results in cardiac depression, which does not occur with the drug administered alone.

2. Ventilation

Morphine causes depression of the respiratory centre, in the medulla oblongata, and this decrease the responsiveness of the respiratory centre to increased levels of carbondioxide. This is because, morphine actson the neurons of the brain stem and decreases the release of the neurotransmitter, acetylcholine, thereby preventing the hypercarbic response. This results in elevated levels of $PaCO_2$ after morphine administration.

The opioid-agonists primarily cause these effects by action on Mu_2 receptor, which is a dose dependent depression of ventilation.

Opioids also interfere with pontine and medullary ventilatory centres, and these leading to prolonged pauses between breathes and periodic breathing.

High levels of opioids will result in apnoea, the patient remains conscious, but is able to initiate and breath when asked to do so. The ventilatory depressant action of opioids, is more pronounced in elderly patients, and who are sleeping.

Opioids cause decrease in the ciliary action, increase in the airway resistance by direct action, and indirectly through release of histamine.

3. Nervous System

Opioids decrease the cerebral blood flow and intracranial pressure. They cause changes, in EEG, which are similar to those evoked by sleep pattern i.e., the rapid a-waves are replaced by the flow of d-waves.

Opioids should not be given to patient of head injury, because,
  (i) It will interfere with wakefulness.
  (ii) Causes miosis
  (iii) Depress ventilation further thus elevating $PaCO_2$
  (iv) Head injury itself causes alteration in blood brain barrier, resulting in increased sensitivity to opioids.

Skeletal muscle rigidity, especially of the thoracic and abdominal muscles, is common with large doses of opioid especially, if administered rapidly. This is due to interaction of opioids with dopaminergic and gamma-aminobutyric acid responsive neurons. Skeletal muscle rigidity, will cause difficulty in ventilation, and if mannual attempts are made to inflate the lung in this condition, will lead to decrease in the venous return. Another cause of inability to ventilater after induction is due to closure of the vocal cords.

Miosis is due to excitatory action of the opioids on the Edinger-Westphal nucleus of the occulomotor nerve.

4. Biliary Tract

Opioids increase the tone of the biliary smooth muscle, resulting in increase in intrabiliary pressure thus leading to biliary colic or epigastric discomfort. The incidence is more with fentanyl. This can be antagonised by administration of naloxone or glucagon (2 mg I.V.) which unlike naloxone, will not severe its analgesic action concentration of smooth muscle of the pancreas, will lead to increases in plasma amylase level and lipase level, which may mimic the picture of acute pancreatitis.

5. Gastrointestinal Tract

Commonly used opioids like morphine and fentanyl cause delayed gastric emptying, by increasing the tone of pyloric sphincters. Also, the propulsive movement in the small and large intestine is reduced, leading to increased water absorption and constipation.

Delay in gastric emptying, increases the chances of aspiration, in anaesthetised patients.

6. Nausea and Vomiting

Opioid induced nausea and vomiting is due to stimulation of chemoreceptor trigger zone in the floor of fourth ventricle, due to its dopamine agonist action.

Morphine

(Figure 2) shows the chemical structure of morphine. Morphine is the gold standard against which all other opioids are compared. It is most commonly used for acute pain in adults and children. It is hydrophilic and does not cross blood brain barrier. It has a poor bioavailability of 20 to 30% which necessitates a large oral dose when converted from parenteral to enteral route. It is used as 10 to 15 mg IM orally and also by IV (10 mg) epidural (3 to 5 mg) spinal route (0.1 to 1 mg). Morphine is metabolised in liver by microsomal mixed function oxygenase that requires P-450 system; metabolising to morphine-6 glucuronide in active form and excreted through kidney. Morphine induces histamine release so used with caution in asthma and allergies. It produces vasodilatation and causes hypotension in hypovolaemic patients. Other side effects are dizziness, constipation, nausea, vomiting, bradycardia, respiration depression, urinaryretention, pruritus, and in high doses myoclonus and seizure. In neonate an immature P-450 enzyme system result in prolonged metabolic rate and higher brain concen-trations and decreased renal clearance seizures 34.

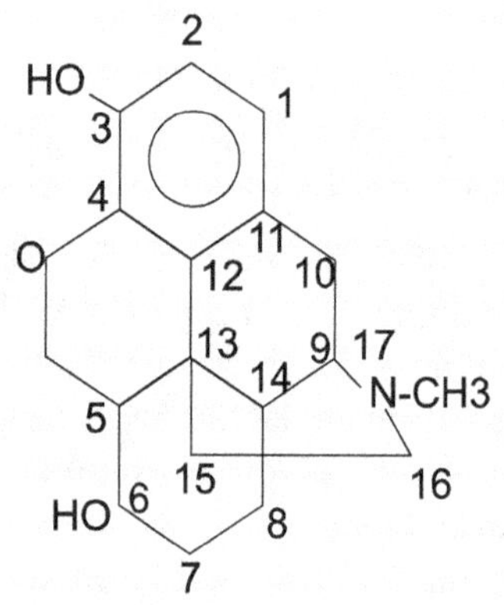

Fig 2: Chemical formula of Morphine

Pethidine

It has one tenth potency of morphine and same drug profile. Its metabolite is normophine with ½ analgesic potency of original base. It interacts with MAO inhibitors in depression. It causes hallucinations, delusions, agitations and seizures. It causes neuroleptic malignant syndrome—hyperpyrexia, acidosis, shock and death.

Butorphanol
Chemical Structure

Butorphanol is a nitrogen substituted 3, 14 dehydrase morphines. N-cyclo butylmethyl group is responsible far the mixed agonist antagonist activity and lipophilicity, whereas the hydroxyl group at C_{14} for additional antagonist activity. The removal of OH at C_6 position also increases analgesic activity.

Mechanisms of Action

Butorphanol is a synthetic opioid, which is a mixed agonist-antagonist.
Butorphanol and its metabolities are agonist at the k-opioid receptor, thereby producing effects like dyspnoea and sedation. It is mixed agonist-antagonist at -opioid receptor, thereby producing effects like euphoria, bradycardia and miosis.

Potency

Butorphanol has been found to be 7 times more potent than morphine, 30 to 40 times more than meperidine and 20 times more than pentazocine.

Pharmacokinetics

The onset of action after I.V. administration is within 10 to 15 sec, with a peak of onset at 0.1 to 1 hr and duration of action, lasting for 3 to 4 hours. It has a half-life of 2.1 to 8.8 hours.

After IM administration, the onset starts at < 10 to 15 minutes with a peak action at 0.5 to 1 hour and duration of action lasting 3 to 4 hour.

Butorphanol is metabolised in the liver chiefly to hydroxy butorphanol, whereas norbutorphanol is produced in small amounts. Since oral bioavailability is only 5 to 17 %, due to high first part metabolism, no oral formulation is available.

The drug binds with plasma proteins, to an extent of 80%. Elimination occurs by urine and faecal route with most (70 to 80%) of the dose is recovered in the urine, and 15% in the faeces. About 5% of the dose is recovered in urine as butorphanol and less than 5% is excreted in urine as norbutorphanol.

The metabolism of the drug through transnasal route is the same as through IM route.

Parenteral butorphanol has been detected in neonatal cord serum with mean neonatal serum concentration, not significantly different from mean maternal serum concentration, following a 1 or 2 mg intramuscular dose. Sedation, is the most common side effect and local effects like nasal irritation and metallic taste are infrequent, so it rapidly course cribriform plate into CNS, neurotoxicity is a potential concern with its cause.

Table 11 : Onset, duration of butorphanol

Parameter	IV	IM
Onset	Rapid	10 –15 min
Peak	0.5–1 hour	0.5 –1 hour
Duration	3 – 4 hours	3.4 hours
Half–life	2.1– 8.8 hours	

Adverse Effects

(i) Cardiovascular: By its action on the Mu receptors, butorphanol can cause hypotension, as observed in < 1%, of the cases, given 1 mg of the drug, through IV route. Similar adverse effect can occur if large doses are administered.

(ii) CNS: Dizziness, confusion, anxiety, exophoria, floating feeling, somnolance nervousness, paraesthesia, abnormal dreams, agitation, dysphoria, hallucinations, lastily, drug dependence.

(iii) Dermatologic: Sweating, rash.

(iv) GIT: Nausea, vomiting, dry mouth.

(v) Others: Lethargy, headache, impaired urination, blurred vision.

Contraindication

- Hyper sensitivity to butorphanol
- Drugs interchange.
- When Butorphanol is used along with CNS depressants like alcohol, barbiturates, tranquilizers, it may result in increased central nervous system depressant actions.

Butorphanol should not be used along with MAO inhibitors and 14 days after administration.

Codeine

Used in oral form in combination with acetaminophen, or aspirin. Causes nausea and allergy. It causes less nausea and vomiting. It has a bioavailability of 60%. Following oral route and plasma half-life of 2.5 to 4 hour with onset of action 20 minutes and duration 60 to 120 minutes. Approximately 120% metabolised to morphine and causes analgesia. Dosage 0.5 to 1 mg/kg. APC contain 12 aspirin acetaminophen, paracetamol and 1 mg codeine per 5 mL. IV injection causes, apnoea, hypotension, histamine release.

Fentanyl

Fentanyl is highly lipid soluble equilibrates rapidly on effector side and has no active metabolites. There is increased clearance in children up to 3 to 12 months of age but a prolonged half life. It can be used IV, IM, SC, transmucosal and transdermal (Duragesic). It is used for short procedures under GA and postsurgical and burns pain relief. It is administered in frequent boluses or continuous IV infusion in 0.5 to 1.0 micg/kg.

Side Effects: Tolerance and dependence by continuous infusion especially in children in ICU.

Sufentanyl

Sufentanyl in 0.25 to 1.0 mcg/kg dose prevents haemodynamic response to laryngoscopy, if given before induction. Maintenance of anaesthetic is achieved with N_2O (60%) and O_2 and intermittent bolus doses of 0.1 to 0.25 mcg/kg. The ED50 of sufentanyl for skin incision is twice as that for intubation is 2.08 mg IV. The ED50 ratios for sufentanyl, fentanyl, and alfentanil in N_2O to O_2 anaesthesia are 1:2:150. Sufentanyl infusions of 1.0 mcg/kg/hr are associated with less postoperative problems. For ventilation 0.25mcg/mL is used.

pKa of sufentanyl is as same as that of morphine (8.0). It is twice as lipid soluble as fentanyl and highly bound (30%) to plasma proteins. It's extractions ratio of (0.8) from liver, means changes in liver flow alters its clearance. It is metabolised by dealkylation, oxidative N-dealkylation, oxidative D-demethylation and aromatic hydroxylation. Major metabolite is N-phenyl piper-amide. It is execrated unchanged in urine due to extensive tubular absorption in kidney.

Alfentanil

Alfentanil clearance (4 to 9 mg/kg) is less than that of fentanyl. It has a long elimination half-life and is less lipid soluble than fentanyl. It is bound to plasma protein at pH 7.4 and it is 90% unionized because of low pKa (6.5). Metabolism occurs by N-alkylation-demethylation aromatic hydorxylation and ether glucuronide. Its major metabolitic is norfentanyl. Others are desmethyl-lalfentanyl, desmethyl fentanil, with little opioid activity. Patients with P-450 3A enzyme activities have low alfentanl clearance.

Doses: 5 to 50mcg/kg used to supplement sedative hypnotic induction or to prevent response to laryngoscopy. Anaesthesia can be maintained with 60% N_2O and O_2 at dose of 0.5 to 2.0 mcg/L/min infusion or bolus of 5 to 10 mcg/kg. Affentanil infusion, should be minimized 15 to 30 minutes prior to end of surgery.

Remifentanil

Remifentanil is a synthetic opioid related to fentanyl congeners; with ester structure, making it susceptible to hydrolysis by blood and tissue non specific esterases, resulting in rapid metabolism. It is a weak base with pKa of 7.07, high lipid solubility, highly bound to plasma proteins (70%). It is unstable in solution so prepared just before use. After IV injection there is a extrahepatic hydrolysis. Its metabolism is by de-esterification for a carboxylic acid metabolite; GI 90291, which depend on renal clearance. Other pathway is dealkylation. It is excreted 90% in urine which are inactive metabolites.

It is administered as a bolus of 1 mcg/kg in combination with propofol for induction of anaesthesia. It can result in hypotension and bradycardia in 10 to 30% patients. So an infusion of

0.1 to 1.0 mcg/min after a bolus is effective, safe, haemodynamically stable, rapid emergence and return.

Table 12 : Opioids intravenous equianalgesic ratio

Drug	Relative Potency	Intravenous loading
Pethidine	0.1	0.5 to 1 mg/kg
Morphine	1	0.05 to 0.1 mg/kg
Methandone	1	0.05 to 0.1 mg/kg
Hydromorphine	5	0.01 to 0.02 mg/kg
Fentanyl	50-100	0.5 to 1mcg/kg
Sufentany	1500-1000	0.025 to 0.05mcg/kg

Referances

1. Kumar P. Textbook of Pain.2nd edition. New Delhi CBS publishers.
2. Miller RD. Miller's anaesthesia. Sixth edition. Elsevier Churchill livingstone. 2729-2786.
3. Healy TE, Knight PR. Wylie and Churchill-Davidson's A Practice of Anaesthesia. Seventh edition. Arnold, London. 1213- 1290.
4. Kumar P.Textbook of Anaesthesia, 2nd Edition. Hyderabad Paras Pub Med.

Chapter 9 Opioid Drug Delivery

Current interest in improving the management of pain by the use of opioid analgesics has led to the search for newer methods of opioid drug delivery. Opioids can be given by (1) sublingual, (2) continuous subcutaneous infusion, (3) transdermal, (4) continuous spinal opioid infusion and (5) intraventricular injection. Each of these modes of administration shares the advantage that they can be used for continuous or repeated administration of an opioid analgesic when injections and oral dosing are to be avoided (table 1). In addition, each of these methods may have advantages in certain therapeutic situations and each mode of administration requires consideration of pharmacological and Pharmacokinetics factors.

Sublingual administration

Although the sublingual route is not a common route of administration for opioid analgesics, it offers a number of potential advantages over injections or the oral route (table 1) the total sublingual and buccal area is small compared to the gastrointestinal tract.

Table 1: Comparison of New Methods of Opioid Delivery[2, 3,4]

Consideration	Continuous Spinal Infusion	Continuous Subcutaneous Infusion	Continuous Transdermal Delivery	Intra-ventricular Injection	Sublingual Application
Avoids im/sc injections	Yes	Yes	Yes	Yes	Yes
Avoids need for iv access	Yes	Yes	Yes	Yes	Yes
Circumvents oral absorption	Yes	Yes	Yes	Yes	Yes
Use by ambulatory	Yes	Yes	Yes	Yes	Yes
Ease of management	Responsible other	Responsible other	Self-administered	Responsible other	Self-administered
Complications	Infrequent but potentially serious	Infrequent, mild	Unknown	Potentially serious	Mild

However, the potential exists for a rapid absorption of drugs in this area is rich in blood and lymphatic vessels. In selecting the opioid that might be suitable for use by the sublingual route, consideration must be given to the principles governing absorption through the oral mucosa and to the physiochemical properties of the opioids (table 2). If the drug is administered in a solid dosage form, then the first step is the dissolution of the dosage form in the tissue fluids (figure 1).

Table 2: Physicochemical Properties of Opioids

Drug	Partition Coefficient *	PKa
Morphine	0.00001	7.9
Hydromorphine	0.0001	
6-Acetylmorphine	0.0012	

Levorphanol	0.01	9.4
Heroin	0.043	
Meperidine	1.7	8.5
Fentanyl	19.68.4	8.4
Methadone	44.6	9.3
Buprenorphine	60.3	

* Heptane and Phosphate buffer at pH 7.4

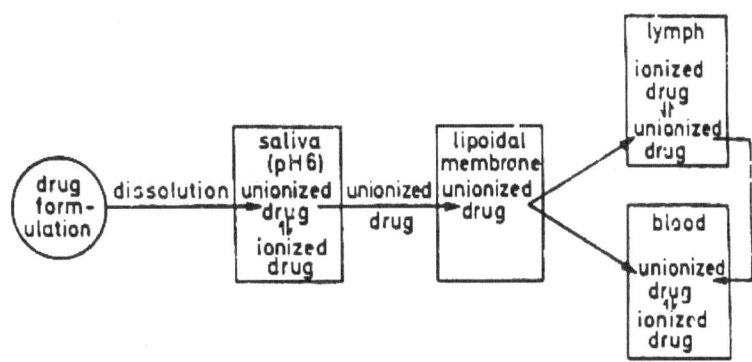

Figure 1: A schematic representation of the sublingual absorption of a drug that is ionized at physiological pH.[4]

The opioids are weak bases and can exist in two forms, an ionized and a unionized form. It is the unionized form that possesses rapidly through lipid membranes into the systemic circulation. The more lipid soluble the unionized form of the opioid, the faster it will be absorbed. As shown in table 2, there are large differences among the opioids in their partition coefficient (PC), an experimentally determined constant that is a measure of lipid solubility. For example, the PCs of methadone and buprenorphine are 6 orders of magnitude larger than the PC for morphine. Indeed morphine is the least lipid soluble of all the clinically used opioids. The order of increasing lipid solubility of opioids (table 2) predicted quite well the order of increasing sublingual absorption. The second important factor is the ionization constant or pKa of the opioid, for it determines the relative amount of ionized and unionized species at a particular pH. The opioids have pKas that vary from 7.9 to 9.4 (table 2) so that by raising the pH of the dosing solution, we can increase the proportion of unionized species of opioid in the sublingual cavity. By control of pH and selection of a lipid soluble opioid, it should be possible to develop opioids, in addition to buprenorphine, that are suitable for sublingual administration.

Patient Controlled Analgesia (PCA)

- Patient Controlled Analgesia (PCA) is a method of pain control that gives the patient the power to control their pain.
  - Pain medication is administered through a computerized pump.
  - The pump contains a syringe of pain medication as prescribed by a doctor that is connected directly to a patient's intravenous (IV) line.
    - The pump is set to deliver a small, constant flow of pain medication.
    - Additional doses can be self-administered as needed by the patient pressing a button.

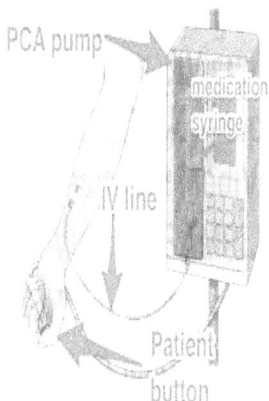

Table 1

Intravenous Opioids for Patient-Controlled Analgesia

Agent	Bolus	Lockout Interval	4 h Maximum Dose	Infusion Rate[a]
Fentanyl (10 µg/mL)	10-20 µg	5-10 min	300 µg	20-100 µg/h
Hydromorphone (Dilaudid) (0.2 mg/mL)	0.1-0.2 mg	5-10 min	3 mg	0.1-0.2 mg/h
Meperidine (10 mg/mL)[b]	5-25 mg	5-10 min	200 mg	5-15 mg/h
Morphine sulfate (1 mg/mL)	0.5-2.5 mg	5-10 min	30 mg	1-10 mg/h

[a] A background infusion rate is not recommended for opioid-naive patients.
[b] Meperidine limit in healthy patients should be 800 mg in the first 24 hours, then 600 mg every 24 hours thereafter. Many institutions limit intravenous meperidine to patients who are intolerant of all other opioids due to safety and toxicity concerns.
Reproduced from [Lennon RL. et al. (2006)[10]].

Continous subcutaneous infusion (CSCI)

Opioids injected subcutaneous in aqueous solution are generally rapidly absorbed with time to reach the maximum concentration in plasma from 10 to 30 min. faster or slower absorption is possible depending on the vascular of the site, the ionization and the lipid solubility of the opioid, the volume of the solution. Opioids, being relatively small molecules, are absorbed directly into the capillaries and the absorption process appears to be limited by blood flow. A prime determinant of the absorption rate from a subcutaneous site is the total surface area over which absorption can occur. Although the subcutaneous tissues are somewhat loose, and moderate amounts of fluid can be administered, the normal connective tissue matrix prevents indefinite lateral spread of the injected solution. The properties shown to be important for the absorption of opioids from the sublingual cavity will also influence subcutaneous absorption.

Coyle et al[5] have evaluated continous subcutaneous infusion of opioids using a portable infusion pump attached to a 27 gauge butterfly needle in the management of pain in cancer pts.

Based on these observations, guidelines for the selection of the opioid and starting dose for CSCI are given in (table 3).

Table 3: Guidelines for Continuous Subcutaneous Infusion (CSSI)
1. Most opioid analgesics available for parenteral use can be administered by CSCI (meperidine [pethidine] and pentazocine are irritating to tissues).
2. May initiate CSCI with the same opioid analgesic that patient have been receiving by the alternate route?
3. Starting dose is calculated using equianalgesic conversing tables (see table 5) with use of rescue doses and titration to effect.
4. Equipment: a portable infusion pump, drug delivery bas, and a 27-gauge pediatric butterfly needle.
5. Home management requires instruction of patient and family.

Table 4: Special Considerations with Continuous Subcutaneous Infusion (CSSI)
1. Local irritation at the site of administration (usually when volume exceeds 1 ml per hour)—more frequent rotation of site infusion
2. Pain breakthrough due to poor absorption from a particular site—change infusion site.
3. Rapidly escalating pain in terminal patients may necessitate the discontinuation of CSCI.
4. Availability of a clinical nurse specialist to assist in home management.

The appropriate management of pts by the use of CSCI requires special considerations as outlined in table 4 and equianalgesic starting doses for some opioid administered by CSCI are given in table 5. these workers found that the steady state plasma morphine concentration varied from 13 to 24 ng/ml during CSCI with a dosage of 2 mg per hour for 12 days in a 22 yr old cancer pt[5].

CSCI has been demonstrated to be a relatively simple, safe and effective method for opioid administration to adults and children in pain. Additional studies are required to continue the development of guidelines of CSCI and determine whether any currently available opioids may possess pharmacokinetic or other properties that make them particularly useful for CSCI.

Continous transdermal delivery

The newest and perhaps most challenging method of opioid drug delivery involves the development of a transdermal drug delivery system (figure 5).

Table 5: Equianalgesic Conversion Ratios[6]		
Opioid Analgesic	Equianalgesic Doses (mg)	
	PO	IM/SC
Morphine	30.0	10.0*
Hydromorphone (Dilaudid	7.5	1.5
Levorphanol (Levo-Dromoran)	4.0	2.0
Methadone	20.0	10.0
* A 1:3 ratio has been used because of repetitive administration		

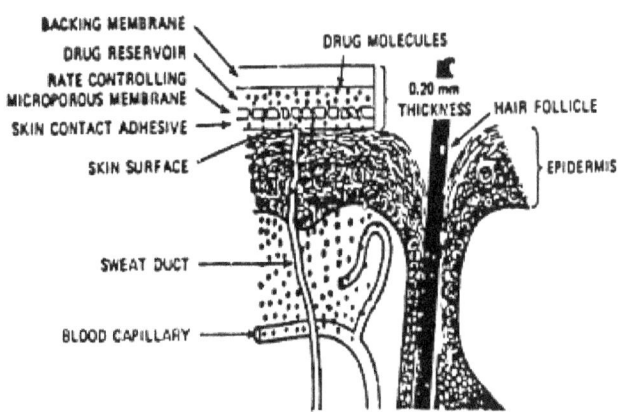

Figure 1: A schematic representation of the flow of drug from a transdermal delivery system through skin into the systemic circulation.

A continous transdermal delivery system for opioid administration offers a number of potential advantages including ease of self- administration (table 1). A critical consideration in the absorption of drugs applied to the skin surface is the properties of the epidermis. This is because despite its thinness the epidermis is a formidable barrier to the absorption of most drugs. Most of the resistance to drug diffusion encountered in the epidermis results from the ultra thin, outermost layer of dead cells called the stratum corneum, the intra cellular space of the corneum contains a unique protein called keratin. Together with a lipid rich medium comprising 15% to 20% of the total stratum corneum, the overall organization is designed to minimize water loss at the body surface. This organization also confers a high resistance to the diffusion of most chemicals. The physiochemical properties of a drug that make it suitable for transdermal delivery are

1. sufficient lipid solubility to penetrate tissue to the capillaries
2. adequate water solubility to allow fairly concentrated solutions (>1.0 mg/ml) to be incorporated into the drug reservoir
3. high relative analgesic potency since it reduces the bulk of the reservoir system.

These considerations have led to the use of the potent, highly lipid soluble opioid, fentanyl in a transdermal delivery system currently under development. Preliminary results indicate that after a lag period of 2-3 hrs, fentanyl appears in plasma and 12 hrs are required for steady state plasma fentanyl levels to be achieved. Additional pharmacokinetic and analgesic studies are required before this potentially useful drug delivery system can be adequately evaluated.

Continuous spinal opioid infusion (CSOI)

Continous spinal infusions of opioids represent relatively a new development in spinal opioid analgesia. Therefore, it is worthwhile to first review the principles and considerations in the spinal opioid analgesia. Spinal opioid analgesia is defined as the introduction of opioids into the epidural or sub arachnoid space for the management of acute and chronic pain. Since its introduction in the late 1970s, it has been used for the management of acute pain in the intra and postoperative period, for obstetrical analgesia and for chronic pain due to cancer and of non-malignant origin[4].

Spinal opioids offer potential advantages over systemic opioid administration including a substantially longer duration of analgesia at much loser dose. Furthermore, if the opioid remains localized to the site of administration then selective activation of spinal cord opioid receptors could provide segmental analgesia without supraspinally mediated adverse affects. Opioid analgesia is free of the sympathetic, motor and proprioceptive adverse effects produced by local anaesthetics. However, adverse effects occur with spinal opioids including sedation, nausea and vomiting, respiratory depression, urinary retention and pruritis[4]. The most feared adverse effect, respiratory depression, occurs as a consequence of rostral redistribution of opioid to supraspinal brainstem sites by movement in the CSF or systemic uptake into the circulation.

Considerable anatomic and pharmacological evidence has accumulated to support the mechanism and site of action of spinal opioids at the dorsal horn of the spinal cord. Opioid receptor densities are the highest in the marginal zone and in the substantia gelatinosa of the dorsal horn. These areas of spinal cord receive primary nociceptive afferent terminals of A delta and C fibers and microinjection of opioids suppresses noxious evoked activity of lamina V neurons. In addition the analgesic effects of intrathecal opioids are dose dependent, stereo specific, antagonized by naloxone and subject to the development of tolerance[7].

Table 6 lists some of the factors that determine the response to spinal opioids. Because of the difficulties involved, few if any controlled studies have compared graded doses of spinal opioids to obtain relative potency estimates. These values are critical for the appropriate comparison among spinal opioids of analgesic time action characteristics and the incidence and severity of adverse effects. it is well established that there are multiple opioid receptor types and that the μ, κ and δ receptor types are to be found in the spinal cord. Currently we lack opioids for use in humans that are highly selective for each of these receptors. However, animal studies have been encouraging[8] and the use of selective opioids and opioid peptides will no doubt improve the specificity of this mode of administration and may overcome the limitations imposed by tolerance.

Table 6: Factors Determining the Response to Spinal Opioids

1. Relative analgesic potency
2. Receptor selectivity
3. Pharmacokinetics in CSF and spinal cord
4. Tolerance to opioids

Table 7: Distribution of Opioids from CSF to Spinal Cord

Opioid	Brain: plasma Ratio	Cord's ratio	Initial Dose in Cord (%)
Morphine	0.046	0.06	3.8
Methadone	1.23	3.1	67.0
Fentanyl	10.58	34.7	95.8

Note: Calculated assuming a cord volume = 10 ml, CSF volume = 15ml, and assuming cord concentration = brain concentration.

Calculations by Bullingham et al[2] predict relatively little uptake of morphine from CSF into the spinal cord at equilibrium (table &). The persistent CSF morphine levels favor redistribution to supraspinal sites. Thus the low lipid solubility and limited uptake into spinal cord of morphine results in a slow onset of action while the slow egress from CSF and spinal cord results in a relatively long duration of action[4]. Furthermore, the supraspinal redistribution of morphine in CSF predisposes to effects mediated cephalad while respiratory movements may enhance the spread of morphine from spinal to supra spinal CSF with pharmacological consequences.

In contrast to morphine, methadone is very lipid soluble (table 2) and is rapidly taken up from the lumbar CSF into the spinal cord (table 7). Rapid egress occurs from CSF leaving a very little methadone available in CSF to move supraspinally (figure 6). Thus lipid soluble opioids such as methadone are characterized by a more rapid onset but a shorter duration of action than morphine. The opioid lofentanil presents a third pharmacokinetic profile. Its lipid solubility is similar to that of methadone resulting in rapid onset but it appears to possess high affinity at μ receptors, resulting in a longer duration of action. increased information on these Pharmacokinetics factors will improve our ability to select the most appropriate opioid for each pt.

Respiratory depression is less common in pts who have developed some degree of opioid tolerance due to prior systemic administration of opioids. Unfortunately the development of tolerance can also significantly reduce the therapeutic efficacy of spinal opioids. Thus, the best time to initiate spinal opioids in pts with chronic pain due to cancer is not yet clear. The difficulties posed by the tolerance development suggest that the chronic use of spinal opioids requires different approaches. Yaksh et al[8] found that in morphine related tolerance rats very little cross tolerance occurs to the delta opioid receptor agonist, DADL, administered intrathecally. Moulin et al[10] found that intrathecal DADL produced safe and effective analgesia in cancer pts with some degree of tolerance to systemic opioids.

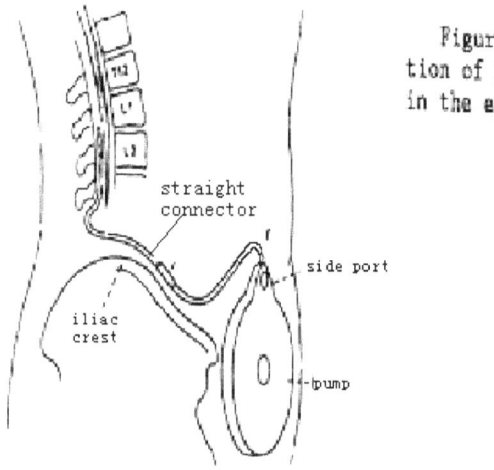

Figure 3 A schematic representation of Infusaid pump with catheter in the epidural space at L1-L2.

Pts with cancer pain require individualization of dose regardless of the route of administration. Cousins and Mather4 have reviewed the use of long-term epidural catheters to administer opioids. Another innovation is a totally implanted system for continous spinal opioid infusion. In addition to the advantages indicated in table 1 CSOI avoids the use of neurolytic agents or neurosurgical procedures for pain control and allows pre operative assessment of the pts response to spinal opioids.

A schematic of the Infusaid model pump 400 is shown in figure 7. The pump includes a 47 ml drug chamber, which is under compression from a temp sensitive bellows. The pump delivers opioid at a constant low rate (2 to 4 ml/day) for 14 to 21 days into a silastic catheter, which is implanted under local, regional and general anaesthesia into the epidural or sub arachnoid space. The pump model also has and auxiliary side port (figure 7), completely by passing the pump mechanisms by implanting the pump in a subcutaneous pocket in the abdomen or chest (figure 8).

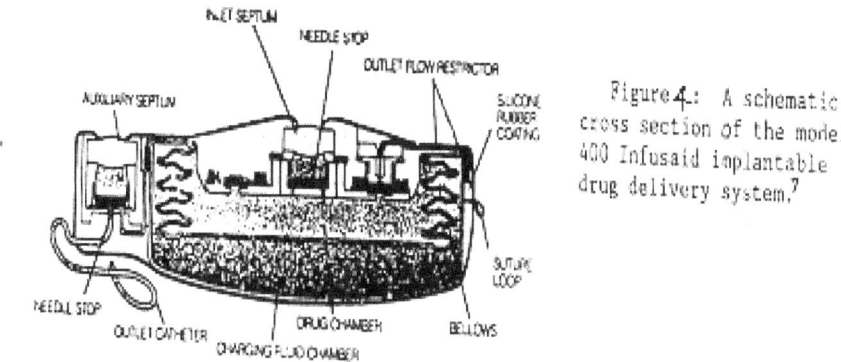

Figure 4: A schematic cross section of the model 400 Infusaid implantable drug delivery system.[7]

However tolerance appears to develop rapidly in some pts and more slowly in others. Tolerance development with or without escalation in pain due to disease progression results in failures after 2-6 months of CSOI. To date, mechanical problems associated with the catheter system and CSF hyromas have been reported. No evidence of catheter induced spinal cord pathology or epidural abscess or meningitis was found in the series[3, 7].

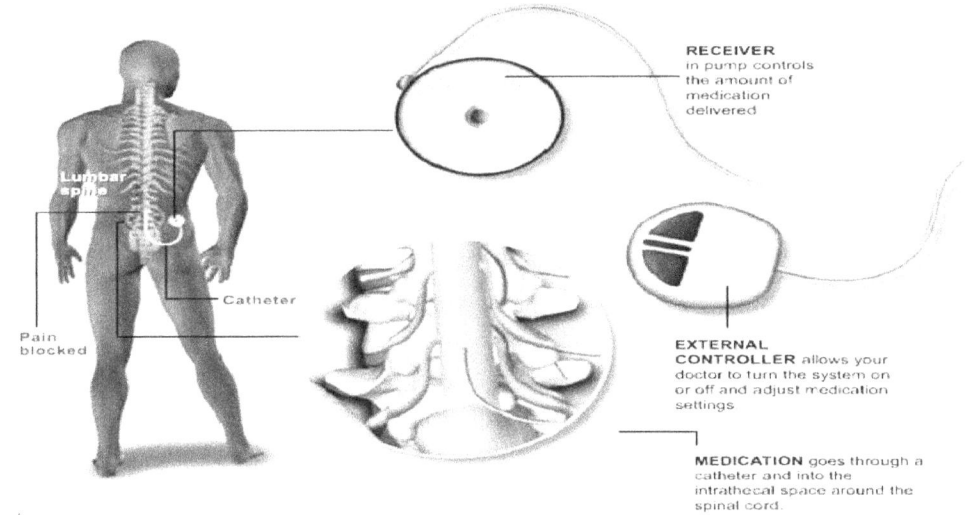

FIG.5. Spinal infusion pump

Smart pumps

Highly sophisticated infusion technology used with both epidural & intravenous infusions. Incorporate multiple comprehensive libraries of drugs, usual concentrations, dosing units and dose limits, to avoid medication errors.

Intraventricular injection

Intraventricular injection of opioid has been reported to be of value in the management of chronic cancer pain. The procedure requires the implantation of an Ommata reservoir to allow IVT opioid administration. The selection of pts and guidelines for the use of IVT are discussed by Lobato et al[11]. table 1 compares IVT administration with the other methods we have discussed. The only opioid used in these reports was morphine in doses that ranged from a starting dose of

0.25 to 1 mg given 1 or 2 times a day[12]. to a maximum dose of 1 to 15 mg given 1 to 3 times per day. Nausea and vomiting occurred in 20% to 60# pts, and other opioid effects including drowsiness and disorientation were reported. The pts developed respiratory depression 4 to 9 hrs after the initial morphine dose. Complications included catheter obstruction and a meningitis, treated successfully with antibiotics. The development of tolerance required a progressive increase in dose. Pharmacokinetic studies confirm very high ventricular CSF levels of morphine, which decay with a t1/2 of 7 hrs[8]. IVT morphine is distributed to cisternal and lumbar CSF[8]. Since opioids can act at spinal and supraspinal sites to produce analgesia, the mechanisms of IVT analgesia may involve multiple sites. It can be assumed that IVT administration of opioids mediate adverse effects such as nausea and vomiting and sedation. It is unlikely that these limitations to the selectivity of IVT administration can be circumvented with available opioids.

References

1. Beckett A.H., Hossie R.D. Buccal absorption of drugs. In: Brodie B.B.,Gillette J.R, eds.,Handbook of experimental pharmacology, vol 28, Springer-verlag, New York, 1971, pp. 25-46.
2. Bullingham R.E.S, McQuay H.J., Moore R.A. Extradural and intrathecal narcotics. In: Atkinson R.S., Hewer C.L., eds., Recent advances in anaesthesia and analgesia, vol 14, Churchill Livingstone, New York, 1982, pp. 141-156.
3. Coombs, D.W., Maurer L.H., Saunders R.L., Gaylor M. Outcomes and complications of continuous intraspinal narcotic analgesia for cancer control pain, J. Clin. Oncol, 1984, 1414-1420.
4. Cousins M.J., Mather L.E. Intrathecal and epidural administration of opioids, Anaesthesiology, 1984, 276-310.
5. Coyle N., Mauskop A., Maggard J., Foley K.M. Continuous subcutaneous infusions of opiates in cancer pts with pain, Oncol. Nur. For., 1986 53-57.
6. Foley K.M. The treatment of cancer pain, N. Engl. J. Med., 1985, 213, 84-95.
7. Greenberg H.S. Continuous spinal opioid infusion for intractable cancer pain. In: Foley K.M., Inturrisi C.E., eds., Advances in pain research and therapy, vol 8, Paven press, New York, 1986 pp. 351-359.
8. Yaksh T L, Achison S R, Durant PAC, Characterisation of action and pharmacology of intrathecally administered DADL encephalin. In: Foley KM Intrurist CE eds. Advances in pain research and therapy, 8, Raven, New York, 1986, 303.
9. Payna R, Interrisi CE. CSF distribution of morphine, methadone and sucrose after intrathecal injection. Life Sci 1986, 37. 1139-1144.
10. Moulin D.E., Inturrisi C.E., Foley K.M. Cerebrospinal fluid Pharmacokinetics of intrathecal morphine sulfate and DADL encephalin Ann. Neurol., 1986, 20, 218-222.
11. Lobato R.D., Madrid J.L., Fatela L.V., Gozalo A., Rivas J.J., Saeabia R. Analgesia elicited by low dose intraventricular morphine in terminal cancer pts. In: Fields H.L., Dubner R., Cervero F., eds., Advances in pain and research and therapy , vol 9 , Raven press, New York, 1985, pp. 673-681.

Chapter 10. Pharmacology of drugs used in Cardiovascular System

Antidysrhythmic Drugs

Cardiac arrhythmias are amongst the most frequent perioperative cardiovascular abnormalities in patients undergoing both cardiac and noncardiac surgery. The mechanism of cardiac dysrhythmia may be different with or without anaesthesia. For example, anaesthetic related cardiac dysrhythmia have been ascribed to abnormal pacemaker activity characterized by suppression of SA node, with the emergence of latent pacemaker within or below the artioventricular tissue. Furthermore, development of rentry circuits is likely to be important in the mechanisms of cardiac dysrhythmias that occur during anaesthesia. Certainly anaesthetics, particularly volatile drugs, may have effect on the specialized conduction system for cardiac impulses [1].

Cardiac antidysrhythmic drugs may be classified on the basis of their electrophysiologic and electro cardiographic effects. The electrophysiologic classification of antiarrhythmic drugs introduced by Vaghun Williams subdivides antiarrhythmics into 4 or 5 classes (Table 1).

Table 1 : Classification of anti-atrhythmic

Class I	Class II	Class III	Class IV
Na^+ channel blocker	b blocker	K^+ blocker	Ca^{++} channel blocker
Ia: Quinidine			
Procainamide	b blocker	Amiodarone	Verapamil
Ib. Lignocaine	Metaprolol	Bretylium	Diltiazem
Mexilitine	Propanolol	Sotalol	
Ic Flecainide			
Eucainide			
Propafenone			

Class I

Drugs in this class interfere with the fast sodium inward current and can decrease the rate of phase of depolarization. As such these drugs may be considered membrane stabilizers.

Class I drugs are further divided into subgroups 1A, 1B and 1C.

IA: Depress phase O depolarization, prolong the action potential duration, and slow conduction velocity.

IB: These drugs shorten the action potential duration and have little effect on phase O depolarization. They depress the conduction of premature beats and conduction through ischaemic tissue.

IC: These drugs markedly depress phase O depolarisation, minimally affect the action potential duration and profoundly slow conduction velocity.

All of the class I drugs depress automaticity, depress conduction in bypass tracts and have depressant effect on phase O depolarization at rapid heart rate.

Class II

The primary action of drug in this class is to suppress adrenergically mediated ectopic activity. They decrease the effective refractory period, action potential duration and automaticity.

Class III

These drugs prolong the duration of the action potential by selectively decreasing potassium ion conduction. Action potential is widened and effective refractory period is increased. They are very effective in prolonging atrial refractoriness.

Class IV

The primary action of this class of drugs is to inhibit Ca^{++} mediated slow channel inward current. Blockade of Ca^{++} channels produces a slowing of conduction and prolonged refractiveness within sinus and atrio-ventricular nodes. The sinus rate decreases, the PR interval is lengthened and there is reduced ventricular response to atrial arrhythmias.

Class V

This class of drugs includes specific bradycardia agent[2]. Alindine has a selective bradycardiac action on the SA node because it reduces the slope of slow diastolic depolarization. The effect may be mediated by a reduction in the chloride current.

Quinidine

It is a class 1A drug, an isomer of alkaloid quinine. It slows down conduction in the bundle of His, decreases the rate of diastolic depolarization and prolongs the effective refractory period, effective in treatment of acute and chronic supraventricular dysrthymias [3].

Metabolism

Quinidine is hydroxylated in the liver to inactive metabolites, which are excreted in urine. As a result of its dependence on renal excretion and hepatic metabolism for clearance from the body, accumulation of quinidine and its metabolite may occur in the presence of impaired function of these organs. (b) Local: Oral candidiasis, hoarseness of voice is common which can be minimised by use of spacer, gargling after use

MAST CELL STABLISER (CROMONES)

The cromones include sodium cromoglycate and sodium nedocromil which prevent the release of inflammatory mediators from various types of cells associated with asthma[3]. They may also have other antiinflammatory actions.
- They stabilize mast cell by preventing calcium entry.
- Pretreatment with these agents inhibits broncho-spasm produced by antigen and exercise. Therefore, these drugs are useful only in the prevention of bronchospasms and not in the treatment of established bronchospasm.

ANALEPTIC DRUGS

These drugs help to restore the drug induced depressed respiratory function toward normal. They block the depressant drug activity either by inactivation or by displacement at the receptor site. The commonly referred analeptic drugs act primarily on the respiratory centres and help to restore the drug induced respiratory depression towards normal. In larger doses, the drugs may stimulate CNS and may even cause convulsions. Some analeptic drugs, indirectly stimulate respiratory centre either through carotid body chemoreceptor (lobeline) or through peripheral sensory receptor (camphor).

Indications of analeptics: Analeptics are useful in hypnotic drug poisoning till IPPV is instituted. Syfocation drawing apnoea in infants respiratory failure during chronic lung diseases and after GA.

Nikethamide

Nikethamide is a sympathetic substance, nicotinic acid diethylamide. It is a cerebral stimulant and an efficient analeptic. It stimulates respiration due to an effect on respiratory centre and not through chemoreceptor of carotid and aortic bodies. It has vasoconstriction effect on the peripheral circulation, with little effect on myocardium but larger doses may increase cardiac output and coronary blood flow. It has a low therapeutic index with a convulsant to respiratory stimulant ratio of 18:1.

Action of nikethamide is usually short, 10 to 15 minutes following IV injection. The usual dose is 1 to 4 mL of 25% solution IV.

Doxapram

Doxapram is a respiratory stimulant. It has a selective effect on peripheral chemoreceptor in the carotid sinus. It stimulates respiratory centre more than the cerebral cortex. It has a wider therapeutic ratio than most other analeptic drugs.

On administration the drug stimulates ventilation and increases cardiac output and work. It can reverse the drug induced respiratory depression. Respiratory stimulation is not usually followed by depression.

Dose: 1 to 5 mg/kg intravenous injection infusion can also be given as 0.2% solution in dextrose at rate of 1.5 to 3 mg/minute.

The drug has brief duration of action only 5 to 10 minutes following a single dose. The drug is rapidly inactivated in the liver, partly metabolized and partly excreted in urine.

Doxapram may be used as adjunct to opiate analgesia, it does not reverse the analgesic effect but can overcome the respiratory depression.

Side Effects

Muscle twitching and convulsion are rare in therapeutic dose. It has a high ratio (70:1), between convulsant and respiratory stimulant dose, in comparison to that of nikethamide (18:1).
During anaesthesia it may induce cardiac arrhythmia. Contraindicated in patient with ischaemic heart diseases or with severe hypertension.
Dosage: Administered mostly orally, 200 to 400 mg three to four times a day.
Intra muscular injection is not recommended because of its associated pain.
It can be administrated intravenous 50 to 75 mg/hr when administration through oral route is unsatisfactory.

Side Effects

Low therapeutic ratio and side effects are predictable if the plasma concentration becomes excessive. As plasma concentration increases 2 mg/mL PR, QRS and Q-T interval increases.

It may cause significant hypotension particularly if administrated IV because of the peripheral vasodilation from alpha adrenergic blockade.

Patient with normal sinus rhythm treated with quinidine may show an increase in heart rate due to anticholinergic action or a reflex increase in sympathetic activity.

Quinidine interferes with normal neuromuscular transmission and may accentuate the effect of neuromuscular blocking drug [4]. Recurrence of skeletal muscle paralysis in the immediate postoperative period has been absent in association with administration of quinidine.

Procainamide

It is an analogue of the local anaesthetic procaine and possesses an electrophysiologic action similar to that of quinidine but produces less prolongation of QT interval on the ECG. Procainamide has no vagolytic effect and can be used in patients with atrial fibrillation to suppress ventricular irritability without increasing the ventricular rate.

Dosage and Route

The drug can be given orally intramuscularly or intravenously usual dose is 0 to 5.1 g, 6 hourly in oral or IM.

Intravenous: 10 to 15 mg/kg loading, 2 to 6 mg/min as infusion.

Metabolism

It is eliminated by renal excretion and hepatic metabolism. In human, 40–60% is excreted unchanged by the kidney, dose must be decreased when renal function is impaired. The major metabolite N-acetyl procainamide has some antiarrhythmic potency.

Side Effects

Hypotension is likely to be caused by direct myocardial depression than peripheral vasodilation.

Ventricular asystole on fibrillation may occur when it is administrated in the presence of heart block, as associated with digitalis toxicity.

Hypersensitivity reaction and systemic lupus erythematosus can also occur.

Lignocaine (XylocaRD, lidocaine)

It is a well known local analgesic agent, used principally for suppression of ventricular dysrhythmia, having minimal effects or supraventricular tachy-dysrhythmia. This drug is particularly effective in suppressing reentry of cardiac dysrhythmia, such as PVC and ventricular tachycardia.

Lignocaine delays the rate of spontaneous phase 4, depolarization by preventing or diminishing the gradual decrease in K^+ ion permeability that normally occur during this phase.

In usual therapeutic dosage, it has no significant effect on either the QRS, QT interval on the ECG. In high doses, it can decrease the conduction in atrioventricular node as well as in the His-Purkinje system.

Dosage and Route

1 to 4 mg/kg loading (over 30 min), 1 to 4 mg/min as infusion.

Decreased cardiac output and hepatic blood flow, as produced by anaesthesia, may decrease by 50% or more in the initial dose.

An advantage of lignocaine compared with quinidine and procainamide is more rapid onset and prompt disappearance of effects when infusion is terminated.

IM absorption of lidocaine is nearly complete. In an emergency situation lignocaine 4 to 5 mg/kg IM, will produce a therapeutic plasma concentration in about 15 minutes. This level is maintained for about 90 minutes.

Side Effects

The principal side effects of lignocaine used to treat cardiac dysrhythmia are neurologic. Stimulation of CNS occurs in a dose related manner with symptoms appearing when plasma concentration > 5 ng/mL.

Seizure at concentration of 5 to 10 ng/mL

CNS depression, apnoea and cardiac arrest are possible when plasma concentration is more than 10 ng/mL.

Mexiletine

It is a long acting lignocaine analogue mainly used to treat dysrhythmia produced by cardiac glycosides and ventricular dysrhythmia after myocardial infarction.

Dose: The usual dose is 200 mg orally 3 times a day.

It may cause hypotension and bradycardia. Adverse effects may involve central nervous system and include nystagmus, ataxia, tinnitus, convulsion etc.

Flecainide

It is an oral antiarrhythmic with an elimination half life 14 hours. It is effective in the control of supra-ventricular tachycardia. However, the drug is arrhythmogenic and the threshold of both defibrillation and ventricular pacing.

Propafenone

It is effective in treatment of ventricular and supraventricular arrhythmias. It has some – blocker activity in addition to class 1C effects. Due to non selective – blocking effect it may exacerbate asthmatic attack.

Class II Agents

Beta adrenoceptor blockers are effective in treatment of arrhythmias caused by increased sympathetic activity. They are also effective in the management of arrhythmias due to a number of factors including increase in plasma catecholamine, leakage of potassium due to hypoxic rise in free fatty acids, and alteration in action potential duration, all of which enhance the heterogenicity of repolarization.

Beta - blockers cause significant reduction in sinus rate and decrease the number of both supraventricular and ventricular arrhythmias [5]. This is associated with a reduction in mortality. – blocker may also reduce the risk of cardiac rupture.

Doses

Propanolol

Usual oral dose for chronic suppression of ventricular dysrhythmia is 10 to 80 mg every 6 to 8 hours.

IV: 1.0 mg/min, can be repeated thrice, if needed over 2 to 3 min interval.

Metoprolol

5 to 15 mg over 20 minutes.

Esmolol

0.5 to 1.0 mg/kg over 5 min, then infusion of 50 to 100 mg/kg/min.

Amiodarone

It is a potent antidysrhythmic drug with a wide spectrum of activity against refractory supraventricular and ventricular tachydysrhythmia[6]. Amiodarone, has non competitive antiadrenergic action, resulting from the inhibition of coupling of β – receptor with the regulatory unit of adenylate cyclase complex. In addition it reduces the density of β adrenoceptors.

The initial dose is 200 mg orally 3 times a day until therapeutic effect is established. Then it is reduced to maintenance dose of 200 mg daily. The intravenous dose is 5 mg/kg given by infusion 20 minutes to 2 hours.

Side Effects

1. Pulmonary toxicity: The most serious side effect is pulmonary alveolitis. It may be because of the ability of amiodarone to enhance production of free oxygen radicals.
2. The drug is an iodinated compound and may disturb thyroid function. Clinical hyperthyroidism or rarely hypothyroidism may occur.
3. Bradycardia, hypotension and even heart block may occur following IV use.

Bretylium

It is generally reserved for the treatment of serious ventricular dysrhythmia that is refractory to suppression with first line drugs such as lignocaine or procainamide.

It has adrenergic nerve blocking activities and accumulates in sympathetic ganglia, decrease noradrenaline release and in high dose cause chemical sympathectomy.

Bretylium is available only for IM or IV administration. The usual dose is 5 to 10 mg/kg IV administrated every 10 to 30 minutes to a maximum dose of 30 mg/kg.

Nausea and hypotension are common after IV administration of bretylium. Conversely, because of initial release of norepinephrine, transient hypertension and increased ventricular irritability may occur after the first few doses.

Class IV

Verapamil

It is a calcium antagonist with a selective inhibitory effect on influx of calcium ions into cardiac cells particularly those of SA and AV node. It is effective in the treatment of intraventricular tachycardia. It is also useful in angina and hypertension as it causes coronary and peripheral vasodilation. Oral dose may be upto 120 mg thrice daily.

IV : 5 to 10 mg IV (75 to 150 mg/kg) over 1–3 minutes followed by a continuous infusion of about 5 mg/kg/min to maintain a sustained effect.

Side Effects

Nausea, dizziness, flushing and constipation. It is contraindicated in patient on b – blockers, disopyramide, quinidine and procainamide, and also suffering from heart block and uncompensated heart failure. (Table 2)

Table 2: Antiarrhythmic drug interactions

Primary drug	Interfering drug	Mechanism	Action
–blockers	Calcium antagonist	Additive cardiodepressant effect	Avoid combined therapy
Digoxin	Diltiazen Quinidine Verapamil	Increased serum digoxin level (mechanism unclear)	Monitor digoxin
Lignocaine	-blocker Cimetidine Barbiturate Phenytoin	Reduced hepatic	Reduced dose by 50%

		clearance Enhanced hepatic clearance	Use high range of recommended doses
Metoprolol	Verapamil	Reduced hypatic clearance	Avoid combined therapy
Procainamide	Cimetidine	Reduced renal clearance	Avoid combined therapy

Diltiazem
It is a benzothiazepine drug with main effect on coronary artery smooth muscle. It has some effect on AV node but little effect on systemic vascular smooth muscle.
Indicated in angina pectoris and Prinzmetal angina.
The usual dose is 180 to 480 mg a day in divided doses.

Adenosine
Adenosine is an endogenous nucleoside that slows conduction of cardiac impulses through the AV-node making it an effective alternative to calcium channel blockers for the treatment of paroxysmal supra-ventricular tachycardia including that due to conduction through necessary pathways in patient of WPW syndrome[17].

Mechanism of Action
It stimulate cardiac adenosine receptors to increase potassium ion current, shorten action, potential duration and hyperpolarize cardiac cells. Usual dose of adenosine is 6 mg IV followed if necessary by repeat injection of 6–72 mg about 3 minutes later.

Side Effects
Associated with rapid IV administration of adenosine includes flushing of face, headache, dyspnaea, chest discomfort and nausea.
It may produce transient AV-heart block.
The pharmacologic effect of adenosine are antagonised by methylxanthines and potentiated by dipyridamole.

HYPOTENSIVE AGENTS
Intraoperative bleeding may be reduced by using locally applied techniques (tourniquets, vasoconstrictions, sympathetic blockade, and posture) or by inducing systemic hypotension. A reduction in bleeding leads to two major benefits, large volume of loses are reduced and the surgical field is improved. Hypotensive agents must be infused through a dedicated line to prevent an inadvertent bolus being given during the administration of another drug.

Infusion should be commenced after the initial response to surgical stimulus has occurred and the infusion rate increased slowly until satisfactory operative condition or a target pressure is attained. Current literature reveals the frequent use of MAP target between 40 and 60 mmHg, with the lower pressure usually reserved for clipping an intracranial aneurysm.

Sodium Nitroprusside (SNP)

Sodium nitroprusside SNP is a direct action vasodilator. The action is due to release of nitric oxide (NO) during metabolism.

It is rapidly degraded by nonenzymatic process in red blood cells and in plasma to release free cyanide (CN), nitric oxide (NO) and methaemoglobin which has affinity for CN molecules to form cyanmethaemoglobin [18].

Administration

Infusion in 0.01 to 0.04% solution. The initial dose is usually 0.2 to .5 mcg/kg per min.

Once prepared the solution must be protected from light as photo degradation of SNP will liberate CN and increase risk of toxicity.

Toxicity

It results in histotoxic hypoxia and systemic acidosis due to inhibition of cytochrome oxidase system. Toxicity is suspected when resistance to infusion and tachycardia persist after the infusion is discontinued.

Pharmacodynamics

CVS

Primarily arteriolar vasodilation has profound effect on both diastolic and systolic pressure.

No effect on heart rate. Sympathetic response is rapid and cardiac output and heart rate may begin to rise within few minutes of starting infusion.

Respiratory

It inhibit hypoxic pulmonary vasoconstriction and increases shunt fractions and V/Q scatter[9]. Alveolar dead space will also rise, if pulmonary perfusion is compromised.

CNS

Sodium nitroprusside (SNP) is a cerebral vasodilator and increases cerebral blood flow and intracranial pressure at normotension[10]. SNP infusion should not be started until the drug is open.

Disadvantages

1. Tachyphylaxis is a serious disadvantage of the drug and is compounded by vasopressin release and after 15 to 30 minutes by an activated renin-angiotensin axis. Angiotension II opposes the action of SNP by direct vasoconstriction and by stimulating release of catecholamines.
2. Ischaemic type EEG changes are more likely with SNP than GTN hypotension[11]. This is probably due to adverse effect that diastolic hypotension has on coronary filling, as well as a steal effect when there is coronary disease.

Glyceryl Trinitrate (GTN)

It is an organic nitrate causing direct relaxation of vascular smooth muscle by reacting with tissue sulphydryl to produce nitric oxide. It is metabolised in liver, RBC and blood vessels, and the active metabolite is excreted through urine. Tolerance to GTN may occur due to saturation of tissue sulphydryl group [12].

Administration

0.01% solution with infusion rate of 10 to 20 µg/min and increased at 2 minute interval to produce adequate control of blood pressure.

Pharmacodynamics
CNS
In low doses it causes vasodilation which results in reflex sympathetic stimulation and in large doses it causes arterial dilation.

Target pressure is achieved slowly and more difficult to maintain with decreased chances of rebound hypertension.

It preserves myocardial perfusion and is the agent of choice in myocardial infarction [11].

Respiratory
It causes pulmonary vasodilation and also inhibits hypoxic pulmonary vasoconstriction response and it increases the shunt and dead space.

CNS
It causes increase in intracranial pressure, less effective in extending lower limit of cerebral blood flow preservation during hypotension.

Toxicity
Acute methaemoglobinaemia may occur and impaired oxygen transport results.

Contraindication
Hypersensitivity to nitrates, severe anaemia, hypovolaemia, preexisting hypotension.

Adequate caution is needed in cases of hypo-thyroidism, hypothermia, malnutrition and liver or renal disease.

Trimetaphan
It is a presynaptic ganglion blockers with a rapid onset of action 1to 3 minutes. Potency is increased by direct vasodilatation and a-adrenergic blockade [13]. It also liberats histamine.

Metabolism
It is metabolised by enzymatic hydrolysis and is partly excreted unchanged in urine which accounts for its short duration of action.

Administration
0.1% solution with a dose of 20 to 50 mg/kg/ min.

Pharmacodynamics
CNS
Primarily arterial vasodilator but vasodilation with blood pooling also occur. Obtunds sympathetic and renin-angiotensin response to hypotension although tachycardia and resistance occur because of vagal blockade and vasopresin release. Rebound hypertension is less common.

Respiratory
Impaired gas exchange by V/Q mismatch, increase bronchial smooth muscle relaxation due to histamine release.

CNS
Little cerebral vasodilation. Intracranial pressure is more stable. Cerebral steal is less likely preferred in presence of focal cerebral ischaemia.

Adverse Effects
Potentiate the nondepoloarizing muscle relaxants and overdose can cause respiratory paralysis [14].

It cause mydriasis because of ciliary ganglionic blockade which prevents the pupils being used as an indicator of cerebral perfusion and anaesthetic depth.

Adenosine

It is a potent vasodilator whose actions are mediated through specific receptors. It has faster onset of action than SNP and with a plasma half life of less than 20 sec, an extremely short duration of action [13].

Features of adenosine induced hypotension are:
- Case of pressure control
- Enhanced cardiac output without troublesome tachycardia.
- Well maintained organ perfusion with a reduction in metabolic demand. Possible analgesic property.
- Minimal tachyphylaxis.

Table 3: Organ effect, doses and kinetics of hypotensive agents[15]

	Nitroprusside	Nitroglycerine	Hydralazine	Trimethaphan
Organ effect				
Heart rate	↑↑	↑	↑↑↑	↑
Pre load	↓↓	↓↓↓	0	↓↓
After load	↓↓↓	↓↓	↓↓↓	↓↓
Cerebral blood ICP flow	↑↑	↑↑	↑↑	0
Kinetics				
Onset	1 min	1 min	5–10 min	3 min
Duration	5 min	5 min	2–4 hours	10 min
Metabolism Blood	Blood, kidney	Blood, liver	Liver	Blood?
Dose				
Bolus	50–100 ng	50–100 ng	5–20 mg	NA
6–12 mg				
Infusion ng/kg min	0.5 to 110	0.5 to 10	.25 to 1.5	10–100 60–120

Effects
- It has potential to cause coronary steal. It is also associated with lactic acidosis and accumulation of phosphate which can potentiate arrhythmias.

ADRENERGIC ANTAGONISTS

Labetalol

It is an adrenoceptor antagonist with actions at α and β receptor. The action at β-receptor is upto seven times greater than that at α-receptor and lasts for 90 minutes as opposite to 30 minutes, found with the later. The overall effect is rapid persistent reduction in blood pressure without concomitant tachycardia with β blockade becomes profound and may lead to bradyarrhythmia or a delay in pressure recovery for several hours.

Dose: 10 to 20 mg intravenous bolus or at a rate of 2 mg/min upto 300 mg. The maximal effect usually occurs by 6 and 5 minutes, after which if goal is not achieved further increments may be given.

Esmolol

It is a β adrenoceptor antagonist with a short half life (of 9 minutes) without tachycardia or rebound hypertension [16]. This is achieved at the expense of myocardial performance and possibly tissue oxygen balance and to be remembered as adjuvant therapy only.

MANNITOL

Mannitol is a derivative of the mannose that does not undergo any metabolism and is rapidly filtered by the glomeruli, leading to osmotic diuresis. It is used as protective and therapeutic agent in neurosurgery or renal compromise and as potential scavenger of oxygen free radicals [17].

Mannitol and Neurocritical Care

The concept of osmotic agents reducing cerebral water content was suggested by Weed and Mekibben in 1919. They noticed cerebral dehydration after intra-venous hypertonic saline [17].

Mechanism for Neuroprotective Effect

1. Osmotic Action: Mannitol is hyperosmolar relative to intracellular fluid hence, intravenous administration result in movement of free water from tissue into the plasma. The blood brain barrier bring relatively impermeable to mannitol, thus maintaining the osmotic gradient.
2. Diuretic Action: Decreases ICP through a fall in CVT as a result of osmotic diuresis.
3. CSF production and reabsorption of mannitol may increase reabsorption and reduce production of CSF by increasing plasma osmolarity. The site of action is postulated to occur at the level of the pial circulation or at cerebral ventricles.
4. **Oxygen free radical scavanger**. Beneficial effect of mannitol could be a reduction of ischaemic damage and oedema by a free radical scavenging action. This may be as a result of specific interference with oedema promoting factors or a reduction in brain tissue necrosis from the primary injury.

Administration

Initial recommended dose of 2 gm/kg has fallen in recent year to between 0.25 to 1 gm/kg and larger dose appear to prolong the effect on ICP.

It should be given by slow bolus infusion over 15 to 30 min to limit significant haemodynamic changesand for repeat bolus it is usually every 3to 4 hours, as this is the time taken for mannitol to clear from circulation if renal function is normal.

Tachyphylaxis may occur with more than 3 to 4 doses per 24 hour complications.

Haemodynamic Changes

Although mannitol increase blood pressure slightly, it can occasionally cause a fall in blood pressure due to a decrease in systemic vascular resistance. The possible cause for this includes a fall in plasma pH, increased release of atrial natriuretic factor, histamine release. Any hypotension is transient but could compromise cerebral perfusion.

Paradoxical Increase in ICP

Any increase in ICP are usually mild and transient and are usually offset by the reduction in brain water and CSF volume.

Dehydration and Electrolyte Disturbances

Dehydration is often concealed as mannitol shifts fluid into the intravascular compartment, thus preserving circulating volume so that clinical signs of haemo-dynamic compromise may not develop until intracellular dehydration is severe. Sodium may increase in the long– term as a result of the hyperosmolar state but is often compensated by an increase in ADH, commonly hyponatremia may also occur due to shift of sodium free intracellular fluid into intracellular space, resulting in dilutional lowering in serum sodium. Rarely, hyper-kalaemia may also occur from haemolysis.

Renal Failure

Mannitol in excess of 200 gm/day may cause acute renal failure.
Hyperosmotality and osmotic compensation

Sustained use of mannitol results in a hyperosmolar state, which lead to movement of osmotically active particles and electrolyte intracellularily. This increase in osmotic activity within all counteract dehydrating effect of hyperosmolar plasma and limit reduction in brain volume. Because of this mannitol should not be used when plasma osmolarity exceeds 320 mOsm/l. Table 4.

Table 4: The approximate osmolarity of mannitol solution

% Mannitol	mOsm/L
5	275
10	550
15	825
20	1110

Mannitol as An oxygen Free Radical (OFR) Scavenger

Mannitol has been proposed to act as an antioxidant OFR scavenger, specifically targeting the oxygen radical, much of the research on mannitol's OFR scavenging capabilities has looked at reperfusion injury, following the restoration of oxygen supply to an ischaemic organ. Cardiac surgery provides one of the easiest models for study in this field. Inspite of cardioplegic solutions and cooling for myocardial protection, there is often some postoperative depression of myocardial function which is thought largely to be due to an excess of OFR produced after cardiopulmonary bypass. Mannitol may act directly to reduce OFR production. It is an effective chelating agent of ferric ion which plays key role in converting poorly reactive oxygen species to highly reactive and damaging oxygen radical.

Other Uses

1. Reduction of intraocular pressure: Mannitol 15-20gm/kg in15/20/25% in 1-15 hrs before surgery.
2. Adjunctive in drug intoxication to promote diuresis : In general, a urinary output of at least 100 mL/hr, but preferably 500 mL/hr and a positive fluid balance of 1 to 2 L should be maintained.
3. TURP: Transurethral restriction of prostate requires irrigating fluid. Solution containing 2.5 to 5% mannitol concentration is used as irrigating solution. Concentration of at least 3.5% is necessary to prevent haemolysis.

Vitamin K

It is a fat soluble dietary principle required for the synthesis of clotting factor. Vitamin K acts as a cofactor at a late stage in the synthesis by liver of coagulation protein–prothrombin, VII, IX and X.

The vitamin K dependent change in these factors confer on them the capacity to bind Ca^{++} and to get bound to phospholipid surface—properties essential for participation in the coagulation cascade.

Daily requirement: It is uncertain because variable amount becomes available from colonic bacteria. Even 3 to 10 mg/kg/day external source may be sufficient. However, the total requirement of an adult has been estimated to be 50 to 100 mg/day.

Deficiency

Deficiency of Vitamin K occurs due to liver disease, obstructive jaundice, malabsorption, long term anti-microbial therapy which alters intestinal flora. The most important manifestation is bleeding tendency due to lowering of the levels of prothrombin and other clotting factors in blood.

Use

The only use of vitamin K is in prophylaxis and treatment of bleeding due to deficiency of clotting factor. In liver disease: associated bleeding responds poorly to Vitamin K because of hepatocellular damage. Synthesis of clotting factors is inadequate despite the presence of vitamin K. However, vitamin K may be of some use if its absorption had been affected due to lack of bile site.

Toxicity

Rapid IV injection of emulsified vitamin K produces flushing, breathlessness, a sense of constriction in chest, fall in BP. It is probably due to the emulsion form of preparation.

Menadione and its water soluble derivatives can cause haemolysis in a dose dependent manner. Patients with G-6-P deficiency and neonates are specially susceptible. In the newborn menadione or its salt can precipitate kerricterus.

(a) By inducing haemolysis and increasing bilirubin load
(b) By competitively inhibiting glucuronidation of bilirubin.

Oxytocin

Oxotocin is a hormone produced by the posterior pituitary. It is also prepared synthetically. It stimulates the contractions of the pregnant uterus both in frequency and magnitude and lays a part in initiating labour [28].

Administration

To induce labour a dilute solution (10 mU/mL) is administered by a constant infusion at 1to 2 mU/min.

Infusion rates of upto 40 mU/minute may be necessary to treat uterine atony, initially after delivery.

Side Effects

Oxytocin in larger doses has a marked but transient direct relaxing effect on vascular smooth muscles. As a result there may be decreasing systolic and particular diastolic pressure, flushing, and increased blood flow in extremities. Oxytocin may cause water intoxication. The dose structural resemblance of the molecule to ADH is responsible for this effect.

Ergometrine

Ergometrine is an ergot alkaloid having a stimulating effect on uterus. The drug acts immediately following intravenous injection and stimulate uterine contraction at all times but is more sensitive in late pregnancy.

It can produce severe hypertension as a result of peripheral vasoconstriction. Ergometrine should be used cautiously when the patient gets another vasopressor drug, otherwise acute pulmonary oedema, cerebral oedema, convulsion may occurs [28].

Administration and Uses

It is used mainly at the end of labour or after caesarean section to produce rapid involution of uterus. It is also used in the treatment of postpartum haemorrhage and atony.

The usual dose is 0.2 to 1 mg or 0.1 to 0.5 mg IV.

The drug is used for in treatment of migraine in dose of 0.5 mg orally.

Phosphodiesterase III inhibitor (PDE III)

Phosphodiesterase III inhibitors inhibit the degradation of cAMP. This increases calcium entry and accounts for the positive inotropic action and has marked systemic and pulmonary vasodilatory effects.

Amrinone and milrinone are the two clinically available PDE III inhibitors.

Milrinone

It has moderately positive inotropic effects with marked pulmonary and systemic vasodilatory effect. It is particularly useful in right ventricular and biventricular failure because of its ability to decrease right ventricular overload.

Milrinone has 20 time more potent inotropic effect than amrinone.

Milrinone improves myocardial diastolic relaxation (positive lusiotropic effect) and decreases left ventricular wall tension, enhancing left ventricular filling and augmenting coronary perfusion.

Dose

Loading dose of 50 mg/kg followed by continuous infusion of 0.5 mg/kg/min.

Amrinone is a PDE III inhibitor

Dose is bolus of 0.75 to 1.5 mg/kg and infusion of 5 to 10 mg/kg/min.

Fenoldopam

Fenoldopam is a DA_1 agonist causing vasodilation by acting on DA_1 receptor in renal, splanchnic vasculature and proximal renal tubule, causing increase in renal blood flow, glomerular filtration rate, naturisis and diuresis.

It also has moderate affinity for a_2 adrenoreceptors.

CVS

It reduces systolic and diastolic blood pressure in patient with malignant hypertension.

Ophthalmic

It causes increase in intraocular pressure, so avoided in patient with history of glaucoma and intraocular hypertension.

Renal

It increases renal blood flow, increases urine flow rate, uterine over sodium secretion.

Onset of action	< 15 minutes
Duration	1 hour
Metabolism	Liver

Dose: Given as a continuous infusion of 0.03 to 0.3 mg/kg/min.

Adverse Effect

Preservative sodium metabisulphate may cause allergic reactions and even anaphylactic reactions.

Anticoagulants

Anticoagulants are drugs that delay or prevent the clotting of blood by direct or indirect action on the coagulation system. The anticoagulants in clinical use are heparin and low molecular weight heparin which is administrated subcutaneously (SC) or IV and coumarin compounds which are administrated orally [19].

Heparin

Unfractionated heparin is composed of a mixture of highly sulphated glycosaminoglycans that produce their anticoagulant effect by binding to antithrombin which is normally present as a naturally circulating anticoagulant. This binding with heparin, however, enhances by about 1,000 times the ability of antithrombin to inactivate a number of coagulation enzymes, including thrombin and activated factors X, XII, XI and IX [19].

Heparin is a poorly lipid soluble, high molecular weight substance that cannot cross lipid barriers in significant amount. As a result, it is poorly absorbed from the GIT and is usually administered by IV or SC injection.

Heparin treatment is usually monitored to maintain the ratio of activated plasma thromboplastin time (APTT) within a defined range of approximately 1.5 to 2.5 times the predrug value, which is typically 30 to 35 seconds.

Heparin effect and its antagonism by protamine are commonly monitored in patients undergoing surgical procedures by measuring clotting time.

Coagulation time (ACT): Because the ACT is easy to use and reliable for high heparin concentrations, it has become the mainstay of heparin anticoagulation monitoring.

Clinical Uses

1. Prophylaxis against venous thromboembolism
   5000 IU SC every 8 to 12 hours.
2. Treatment of venous thromboembolism
   5000 IU IV followed by continuous infusion of 30000 U every 24 hours.
   The goal is to maintain the APTT at 1.5 to 2.5 times the laboratory control value.
3. Treatment of unstable angina and acute myocardial infarction.
   5000 U IV of heparin followed by infusion of 24000 U every 24 hours.

Side Effects

1. Haemorrhage
2. Thrombocytopenia
3. Allergic reaction
4. Hypotension
5. Altered protein binding
6. Decreased antithrombin concentration.

Low Molecular Weight Heparin (LMWH)

Enoxaparin is LMWH derived from standard commercial-grade unfractionated heparin by chemical depolymerization to yield approximately one-third the size of heparin [20]. These fragments are heterogenous in size, with a mean molecular weight of 4000 to 5000 daltons.

Depolymerization of heparin results in a change in its anticoagulation profile, pharmacokinetics and effects on platelet function. Enoxaparin exhibits less binding to endothelial cells than does heparin, a property that accounts for its longer elimination half time that permits once daily dosing without laboratory monitoring.

Protamine

Protamine is the specific antagonist of heparin's anticoagulant effect. It is strongly alkaline polycationic low molecular weight potein found in salmon sperm. The positively charged alkaline protamine combines with the negatively charged acidic heparin to form a stable complex that is devoid of anticoagulant effects. These heparin protamine complexes are removed by reticulo endothelial system.

The dose of protamine required to antagonize heparin is typically 1 mg for every 100 U of heparin predicted to still be circulating.

Adverse cardiovascular responses to protamine include hypotension, pulmonary hypertension and allergic reactions.

Hexadimethrine: It is the only drug alternative to protamine.[21]

Oral Anticoagulants

Oral anticoagulants are derivative of 4-hydroxy coumarin[32]. The essential chemical characteristics of coumarin derivatives for anticoagulant activity are an intact D. hydroxy coumarin residue with a carbon substitution at the number 3 position (Table 5).

Table 5: Comparison of anticoagulant drugs

Anticoagu-lant drug	Time to Plate effect (hr)	Duration after discontinuation	Dose Initial (mg)	Main-tenance
Warfarin	36–72	2.5	15-first day 20 second	2.5 to 10

Dicoumarol	36–48	2–6	200–200 first day	25–200
			10 third day	
Phenindione	18–24	1–2	300 Ist day 200	25–200

Mechanism of Action

Warfarin inhibits vitamin K epoxide reductase and thus blocks the conversion of vitamin K epoxide to vitamin K. Subsequent depletion of vitamin K results in production of haemostatically defective vitamin K dependent coagulation protein. Platelet activity is not altered by oral anticoagulants.

For most indications modulate anticoagulant effect with a targeted international normalized ratio (INR) of 2.0 to 3.0 is appropriate.

Management before Elective Surgery

Relatively minor surgical procedures can be safely performed in patients receiving oral anticoagulants. For major surgery, discontinuation of oral anticoagulants 1 to 3 days preoperatively is recommended to permit the prothrombin time to return to within 20% of its normal range [23].

In emergency situations, IV administration of vitamin K, fresh whole blood or fresh frozen plasma may be necessary to abruptly counter the effects of oral anticoagulants.

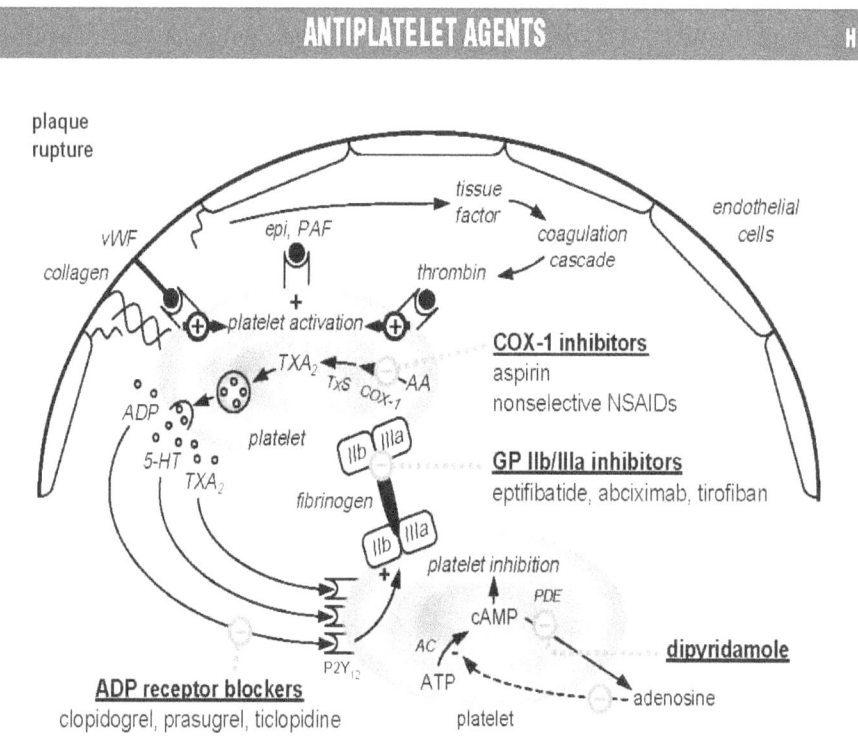

References

1. Atlu JL, Bosnjak ZL. Mechanism of cardiac dysrrhythmias during anaesthesia. Anesthesiology 1990;72:347–74.
2. Kobingen W. Specific bradycardiac agent. In: Vaughan William Em ed. Antiarrhythmic drugs Berlin: Springervurlag 1989:423–52
3. Grace AA, Camm AJ. Quinidine. N Engl Mid 1998; 338:34–45.
4. Harrah UD, Way WL. The interactions of d tubocurarine with antiarrhythmic drugs. Anesthesiology 1970;33:406–410.
5. Rossi PRF, Ysul S. Reduction of ventricular arrhythmias by early intravenous atenelol in suspected acute myocardial infarction. British Medical Journal 1983;286:506–10.
6. Singh BN, Chew CYC. New perspectives in the pharmacologic therapy of cardiac arrhythmias. Progress in Cardiovascular Disease 1980;22:243–301.
7. Lerman BB, Belardinelli. L Cardiac electrophysiology adenosine basic and clinical concepts. Circulation 1991;83:1449–1455.
8. Skoda S, Frank PA, Homan SM In viro cyanide release from sodium nitroprusside Anaesthesiology 1987;66:381–5
9. Cschely pA, Lear S, Cottrell JE. Intra pulmonary shutting during induced hypotension Anesthesia and Analgesia. 1982;61:231–5.
10. Turner JM, Powell D. Intracranial pressure changes in neurosurgical patients during hypotension induced by sodium nitroprusside or trimestaphan. British Journal of Anaesthesia 1977;49:419–24.
11. Blood BC, Mal et al. Myocardial haemodynamics during hypotension: A comparison between SNP and Adenosine Anaesthesia 1978;49:17–20.
12. Needlam P, Johnson EM. Mechanism of tolerance development to organic nitrates. Journal of Pharmacology 1973;184:709–15.
13. Fahmy NIR, Soter NA. Effect of Trimethapan as arterial vasodilator and a-adrenergic antagonist. Anesth and Analg 1984;63: 290–15.
14. Dale RC, Schroeder ET. Respiratory paralysis during treatment of hypertension with Trimethapan. Archives of Internal Medicine 1976;136:816–18.
15. Laing BT. Adenosine receptors and cardiovascular functions. Trends in cardiovascular medicine 111992;2(3):100–8.
16. Khambatta HJ, Stone JG, Khan E. Propanolol premedication-blunts stress response to nitroprusside hypotension. Anesth Anal 1984;63:125–8.
17. Healy TEJ, knight PR (Ed). Churchill-Davidson A practice of Anesthesia, London, Arnold, 2004.
18. Miller J. Anesthesia 6th Ed. Philadelphia, Churchill-Livingstone, 2004.
19. Hirsh J. Heparin. N. Engl. J Med. 1991a;324:1565–73.
20. Weitz JI. Low molecular weight heparin. N Eng J Med 1997;337:688–98.
21. Kikura M,Lee MK, Heparin Neutralization with methylene blue, hexadimethrine or vancomycin after cardiopulmonary bypass. Anesth Analg 1996;83:233–27.
22. Hirsh J. Oral anticoagulant drugs. N Engl J Med 1991b;324:1865–75.
23. Tinker JH, Tarshan S. Discontinuity anticoagulant therapy in surgical patients with cardiac value prosthesis. JAMA 1978;239:738-40.

Chapter 11. Respiratory and Adjuvant Drugs

RESPIRATORY SYSTEM

Bronchial smooth muscles are innervated with both sympathetic and parasympathetic fibres. Sympathetic fibres by liberating catecholamines at postganglionic nerve ending cause bronchodilation. Para sympathetic stimulation and sympathetic blockade causes broncho-constriction[1].

Asthma is the most common chronic pulmonary disease with a global incidence of 3 to 7%. It is an inflammatory disease of airway with reversible expiratory airflow obstruction [2]. High mortality is due to ineffective or inadequate treatment leading to irreversible changes in the airway. Patients who have increased airway responsiveness and therefore, are candidates for preoperative bronchodilation are smokers, a topic symptoms of allergies [3], patients with COPD and asthmatics.

Drugs used for treatment of bronchial asthma
1. **Bronchodilators**
   A. **Sympathomimetics**
      Adrenaline, Ephedrine, Isoprenaline, Salbuta-mol, Terbutaline, Salmetrol.
   B. Methylxanthines
      Theophyllines, Aminophylline, Choline theo-phyline.
   C. Anticholinergics
      Atropine methonitrate, Ipratropium bromide, Tiotropium bromide.
2. **Mast Cell Stablizers**
   Sodium crommoglycate, Nedocronic, Ketotifen.
3. **Corticosteroids**
   A. Systemic: Hydrocortisone, Prednisolone.
   B. Inhalational: Beclomethasone dipropionate, Buclesonide, Flunisolide, Triamcinolone, Fluticasone, propionate

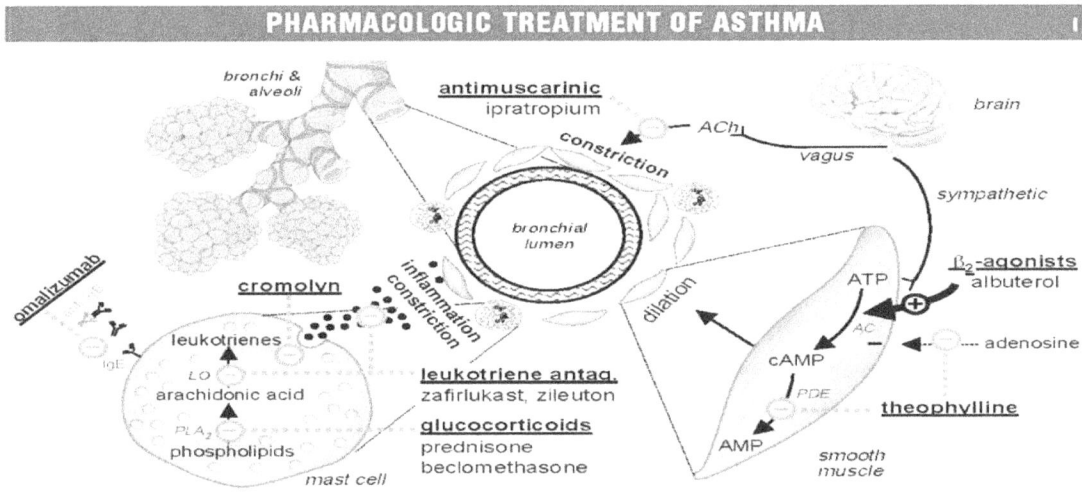

Fig 1: Mechanism of action of anti asthmatic drugs.

Sympathomimetics

Adrenergic drugs cause bronchodilation through β receptors stimulation. They act on the target cells in the lung by increasing the activity of adenyl cyclase, an enzyme in the cell membrane which catalyses the formation of cAMP from ATP. cAMP functions as a second messenger in the cell where it acts on the smooth muscle to decrease tension and motility. In addition, adrenergic compounds (epinephrine ephedrine, isoproterenol) can also increase ciliary activity, this may help in removing secretions[4] (Table 6).

Table1: Drugs used for treatment of bronchial conditions

Drugs	Action	Dose
Adrenaline	α, β and β$_2$ agonist causes short lasting Bronchodilation	
Ephedrine	α, β, β$_2$ action Slow developing Bronchodilation lasting from 3-5 hours	
Isoprenaline	β$_1$ and β$_2$ agonist causes prompt Bronchodilation, lasting from 1-2 hours	10-20 ng SI 1-2 mg IM .4 to 8 mg inhaled
Orciprenaline	Somewhat selective β$_2$ agonist 0.65 to 1.3 mg Longer acting 3-4 hours	20 mg oral 0.5 to 1 mg IM/Sc by inhalation
Salbutamol	β$_2$ agonist Highly selective longer acting and Safer than isoprenaline by inhalation	2-4 mg oral .25 to .5 mg IM/SC 100-200 mg
Tarbutaline	-do-	5 mg oral .25 mg sc 250 mg by inhalation
Salmeterol	Long acting selective β$_2$ agonist	25 mg/MDI 2 puffs BD with a slow onset of action

Adrenergic drugs are the mainstay of treatment of reversible airway obstruction. Should be used continuously in hypertensives, heart patients and in those receiving digitalis.

They are the fastest acting when inhaled.

- Adrenergic drugs are the mainstay of treatment of reversible airway obstruction.
- Should be used continuously in hypertensives, heart patients and in those receiving digitalis.
- They are the fastest acting when inhaled.
- Side effects due to the stimulation of adrenergic receptors in the cardiovascular system are more common with mixed agonist, but it may occur with selective beta $_2$ agonist, specially at higher doses.

Methylxanthines

Caffeine, theophylline and theobromine also cause bronchodilation by increasing cAMP but by a mechanism different from that of b_2 adrenergic receptor agonists cAMP is broken down by cytoplasmic enzyme, phosphodiesterase whose activity is inhibited by methylxanthines such as theophylline and aminophylline (Fig.2).

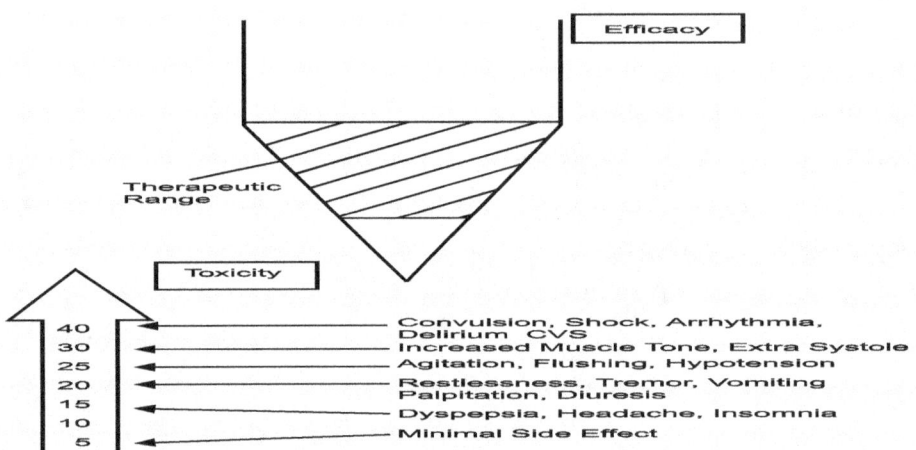

Fig. 2: Therapeutic range and toxicity of methylxanthines.

- Because methylxanthines and $_2$ agonist act by different mechanism, theophylline is often given to patients with bronchospasm already receiving agonist, and thus they work in synergy to increase intracellular concentration of cAMP [5].
- In addition, aminophylline improves the contractility of the diaphragm and renders it less susceptible to fatigue [6].

Pharmacological Actions

1. CNS: They stimulate medullary, vagal respiratory and vasomotor centre. Vomiting at high doses is due to both gastric irritation and CTZ stimulation.
2. CVS: Directly stimulates the heart and increase forces of myocardial contraction. Tachycardia is more common with theophylline but caffeine generally decreases heart rate.
3. Smooth muscles: All smooth muscles are relaxed. The action is direct as well as due to release of and may be potentiation of adrenergic trans-mitter.
4. Kidney: Mild diuresis; acts by inhibiting tubular reabsorption of Na^+ and water.
5. Stomach: Enhance secretion of acid and pepsin. Also gastric irritant.

Interactions

(a) Drugs which inhibit theophylline metabolism and increase its plasma level are: erythromycin, cipro floxacin, oral contraceptives; doses should be reduced to 2/3rd.

(b) Theophylline enhances the effect of furosemide, sympathomimetics, digitalis, oral anticoagulant.

(c) Theophylline decreases the effect of phenytoin, lithium.

- The bronchodilation activity of oral theophylline is relatively weak and high doses are needed. Lower doses of theophylline show antinfla-mmatory effect which make it an important drug for the treatment of asthma. It is poorly water soluble, cannot be injected. Dose 100–300 mg TDS.
- Aminophylline: Though popular than theophy-lline due to better solubility with the addition of solvent ethylenediamine but has a lower theurapeutic index. Therefore, it should be administered very cautiously preferably with ECG monitoring.
  Usual intravenous loading dose is 5 mg/kg IV slowly followed by continuous infusion of 0.5 mg/kg mixed with dextrose solution.

ANTICHOLINERGICS

- Cause bronchodilation by blocking cholinergic constrictor tone. However, they are less efficacious than sympathomimetic, but can add to their response.
- Patients with asthmatic bronchitis, COPD and psychogenic asthma respond better to anti-cholinergics.

• Inhaled anticholinergics produce slower response than inhaled sympathomimetics and are better suited for regular prophylactic use than for control of an acute attack.

Corticosteroids

These drugs are the most effective antiinflammatory agents in treating asthma. They act in a relatively nonspecific manner by inhibiting a variety of infla-mmatory cells, cytokine expression and transcription factors which are involved in the inflammatory disease process [7]. They also increase the number of the β– receptors and thus may increase the sensitivity of $β_2$– receptor agonist [8].

By inhalation of corticosteroid a higher concentration of steroid can be achieved in the airway while minimising the side effects associated with the systemic administration. These topical steroids have high local anti-inflammatory potency due to high affinity for glucocorticoid receptor, with low systemic side effects due to poor absorption and rapid inactivation byliner [9].

- Peak effect is seen after 4 to 7 days of instituting inhaled steroids and benefits for a few weeks after discontinuation.
- Patient on oral steroid should receive inhaled steroid in addition, for 1to 2 weeks before the former is tapered, otherwise steroid withdrawal may manifest. This confirms each of systemic activity of inhaled steroid (< 100 mg/day)

(a) Systemic: Adrenal suppression[10], osteoporosis, growth suppression cataract.
   It should not be used in cases with thyrotoxicosis and status asthmatics.
  Contraindicated in patients with ischaemic heart disease or with severe hypertension.
  It should not be used in cases with thyrotoxicosis and status asthmaticus.
  Ethyl and propyl butamide (Micoren) A solution containing equal amount of the two is available. Dose-100 mg in oral perls, drops and 200 mg/1.5 ml injection. It is not used presently in anaesthesia practice

ANTIEMETIC DRUGS: Vomiting is a protective reflex mechanism to protect the body from toxins ingested in food. Nausea and vomiting

Mannitol and Renal Protection

Mannitol is effectively inert and is freely filtered at the glomerulus without being secreted or substantially re-absorbed (< 5%). Diuresis is best with total body water loss upto 30% of filtered amount. The precise mechanisms by which the diuresis occurs have not been fully elucidated, but include changes of systemic and renal haemodynamics as well as local effects at the glomerular and tubular levels.

Systemic Haemodynamic Changes

Following intravenous administration, mannitol is confined mainly to intravascular compartment causing a water shift from intravascular compartment, which cause intravascular volume expansion and decreased plasma oncotic pressure, blood viscosity and haematocrit, all of which may improve renal perfusion.

Renal Haemodynamic Effects

Infusion of mannitol has been shown to improve renal blood flow (RBF) and glomerular filtration ratio (GFR) by reducing renal vascular resistance (RVP). Increased renal perfusion is associated with proportional increase in cortical and medullary blood flows. Conversely, high doses of mannitol may cause renal artery vasospasm and increased RV resulting in decreased renal perfusion, which may paradoxically impair renal function.

Glomerular Effects

Mannitol has been shown to restore GFR of a hypoperfused kidney to near normal values. Mechanism proposed includes preferential dilatation of the afferent glomerular arteriols due to suppression of renin release and intrarenal formation of angiotension II.

Tubular Effects

Mannitol is completely filtered at the glomerulus. Without any reabsorption and as a result, there is increase in osmolarity of renal tubular fluid and this prevents reabsorption of water. Sodium is diluted in this retained water in the renal tubules, leading to less reabsorption of this ion. Hence along with the osmotic diuretic effect, there is urinary secretion of water, sodium, chloride and bicarbonate ions.

Renal ischaemia of whatever origin leads to tubular cell oedema. This comprises the interstitial and vascular spaces, resulting in poor renal perfusion and impaired renal function. Mannitol has been shown to reduce tubular cell swelling, particularly in the proximal tubule and thick ascending limb of the loop of Henle and it is assumed to maintain both tubular flow and glomerular filtration.

Mannitol increases both renal blood flow and glomerular filtration and thus there is a greater solute and water load to be reabsorbed by the tubules. This leads to energy expenditure and a concomitant rise in oxygenmay also be induced by irritation or distension of upper GIT, distension of duodenum being particularly strong stimulus[28].

Dopamine antagonists are mainly used in severe chemotherapy induced emesis suggesting no dopa-minergic emetic mechanism involved (Table2).

Table 2: Dopamine antagonists used in PONV

Drug	Mode	Elimination half–life	Adverse effect
Droperidol	IV and IM	2 hours	Extrapyramidal disorder (EPD) Delayed recovery Hypotension Anxiety
Prochlorpera-zine	IV and IM	6–8 hours	EPD Delayed recovery

Metaclopramide	Oral, IV	4 hours	EPD
IM			Restlessness
Domperidone	Oral and rectal		Cardiac dysrhythmic

Granisetron

Granisetron, α 5-HT₃ receptor antagonist was introduced for the prophylaxis and treatment of chemotherapy and radiation induced emesis, but are also used to treat postoperative nausea and vomiting. It has no effect on gastric emptying or on small intestine transit, but does delay colonic transit.

Table 3: Neurotransmitter involved in nausea and vomiting

Dection of emetic stimulus	Stimulus	Neurotransmitter	**Receptor**
Afferent input from GIT	Irritation and distension	5 HT Substance P	5HT3
Area posterna (CTZ)	Toxin and chemicals	Dopamine	D_2
Vestibular nuclei	Motion	Acetylcholine histamine	Muscarinic H1
Vomiting or emetic centre	Input from other area	Acetylcholine histamine substance P	Muscarinic H_1 NK_1

Dose: An intravenous dose as low as 0.04 mg/kg is effective in prevention of PONV.

The elimination half-life of granisetron is 2.5 times longer (9 hours) than that of ondensetron and this may require less frequent dosing.

Metabolism

The drug is rapidly and extensively metabolised in liver, 12% of the administrated dose of the drug is eliminated unchanged in the urine.

Contraindications

In patient with subacute intestinal obstruction and in patients with history of hypersensitivity.

Ondensetron

Dose: 0.06 mg/kg IV.

References

1. Shepherd IN. Postoperative intensive care of patients with respiratory disease. International Practice of Anaesthesia. Oxford. Butterworth 1996:1/68/1–17.
2. Horwitz RI, Busse WW. Inflammation and asthma. Clin Chest Med 1982; 16:126–35.
3. O' Cornea G, Segal MR, Weiss ST. Smoking, atogcy and metacholine airway responsiveness among middle aged and elderlymen. The normatine aging study. Am Rev Respi Dis 114:1145;1976.
4. Mullmille GN, Irnani J. Adrenergic compound and respiratory tract. A physiological and electronic microscopal study. Respiration 33:261;1976.
5. Webb-Johnson DC, Cher B. Bronchodilator therapy. N Engl J Med 297; 476:1977.
6. Aubiur M, Sampson M et al. Aminophylline improve diaphragmatic contractility N Engl J Med 305;249:1981.
7. Barnes PJ, Pedersen S. Efficacy and safety of inhaled corticosteroid new developments. Am J Respir Crit Care Med 1998;157:511–53.
8. Frasen CM, Venter JC. Beta-adrenergic receptors: Relationship of primary structure, receptor function and regulation. Am Rev Respir Dis 1990; 1141; 522–535.
9. Toogood JH. Complication of topical steroid therapy for asthma. Am Rev Respir Dis 1990; 141:589–92.
10. Boosma M, Andersson N. Assessment of relative systemic potency of inhaled fruitcasome and budesomide. Ein Respir J 1996;9:1427–32.

CHAPTER 12. CENTRAL NERVOUS SYSTEM

ANTIPSYCHOTIC DRUGS
- Primary effects on psyche.
- Useful in all types of psychosis especially schizophrenia.
- Also could be neuroleptic, ataractic, major transquillizers.

Table 1: Antipsychotic drugs[1]

Classification	Drugs
1. Pheno thiazenes	
Aliphatic side chain	• Chlorpormazine
	• Triflupromazone
Piperadine side chain	• Thioridazine
Piperzine side chain	• Trifluperazine
	• Fluphenazine
2. Butyrophenones	• Haloperidol
	• Droperidol
	• Trifluperidol
	• Penfluridol
3. Thioxanthenes	• Thiohexine
	• Tflupenthixol
4. Heterocyclics	• Pimozide
	• Loxapine
	• Reserpine
5. Other neuroleptics	• Clozapine
	• Olanzipine

Pharmacological Actions

1. CNS
- Aliphatic and piperidine side chains—low potency and more sedative action.
- Tolerance to sedative action develops over weeks, but not to antipsychotic action.
- Extrapyramidal side effects most common with high potency drugs, is least with thioridazine more with trifluperazine, fluphenazine.
- Chlorpromazine lowers seizures threshold, can precipitate in untreated epileptics.
- Temperature control is knocked off at higher doses, respiratory and medullary centres are affected in the end.
- Except Thioridazine, all are good antiemetic, action expected through CTZ.
- In normal individuals, the drugs calm the subjects, cause indifference to surroundings, cause paucity of thoughts, psychomotor slowing emotional quietening and tendency to go off to sleep without being arousable.

Mechanism of Action: Dopamine 2 (D_2) receptor blocking action, in the temporal and prefrontal areas, constituting the limbic system and in mesocortical areas.
- Initially, as an adaptive change the dopamine (DA) neuronal firing and DA increases but later on it diminishes, especially in basal ganglia giving rise to extrapyramidal effects.
- DA blockade in CTZ produces antiemetic action.
- Clozapine and olanzipine act by blockade of $5-HT_2$ and $beta_1$– receptors.

2. ANS (Autonomic Nervous System)

Chlorpromazine (CPZ)
- bet-adrenergic blocking activity.

CPZ = Triflupromazine > thioridazine.

> fluphenazine > haloperidol
> trifluperazine > clozapine
- Anticholinergic property is graded as:
  Thoridazine > chloroppromazine
  > Triflupromazine = haloperidol
- Olanzipine is potent anti muscaranic.

3. Local Anaesthetic
Chlorpromazine has local anaesthetic action but not used as it is irritant.

4. CVS
- By central as well as peripheral action cause reflex tachycardia
- Not seen in psychotics
- Accentuated by hypovolaemia.
- Tolerance develops to hypotension.
- Myocardial depression at high doses of CPZ chlorpromazine prolongation of AT interval.

5. Skeletal Muscles
They decrease certain types of spasticity.

6. Endocrine
- Inhibits DA in pituitary, causes protectin release and leads to galactorrhoea, gynacomastia.
- ACTH response to stress is diminished.
- Decrease ADH increase in urine volume.

Tolerance and Dependence
Tolerance to sedative and hypotensive effect in days or weeks. No dependence.

Pharmacokinetics
Oral effects of CPZ are unpredictable, more consistent effects with IV or IM injection.
- Bound to plasma proteins, and metabolized by the liver.

Adverse Effects
(i) CNS: Lethargy, sedation, mental confusion, tolerance develops, precipitates seizure in uncontrolled epileptics.
- Clozapine and olanzipine can induce seizures.

(ii) b –blockade: Palpitation, hypotension, difficulty in ejaculation, more with thoridazine.

(iii) Anticholinergic: Dry mouth, blurring of vision, urinary hasitancy, constipation. Clozapine causes hypersalivation.

(iv) Endocrine: Galactorrhoea, gynecomastia.

(v) Extrapyramidal effects:
- Dose limiting side effects.
- Common with high potency drugs pimozide, fluphenazine, haloperidol.

(a) **Parkinsonism**: Rigidity, tremors, hypokinesia, mask like face, appears in 1 to 4 weeks.

(b) **Acute muscular dystonia**: Bizarre muscle spasm involving linguo-fascial muscle grimacing, torticollis, locked jaw, after few hours or 1st week of therapy. Common in children < 10 years, more in girls, after parenteral administration. Central anticholinergics, like promethazine IM clears the reaction in 10 to 15 minutes.

(c) Restlessness, apparent agitation, feeling of discomfort (1 to 8 weeks).
- Addition of diazepam may help.

(d) **Malignant neuroleptic syndrome**
- Rare with high doses of potent neuroleptics appears in 24 to 72 hours.
- Marked rigidity, immobility, tremors, fever, semi consciousness, fluctuating BP and HR, myoglobin may be present in blood.
- Lasts 5 to 10 days after withdrawal of the drug, may be fatal.
- Intravenous dantrolene may help.

- Bromotriptine in large doses is useful. Due to dopamine blockade in hypothalamus and basal ganglia brain stem. Loss of thermal regulation.

  (e) **Tardive dyskinesia**

  It is characterized by purposeless involuntary movements, of face and limbs, like chewing, ponting, lip-smooking, puffing of cheeks.
- Common in elderly women, due to neuronal degeneration.
- Accentuated by anticholinergic.
- Occur in 10 to 20% cases, may subside in weeks, months or may be lifelong.

(vi) Hypersensitivity reaction

Cholastatic jaundice (phenothiazine) skin, rashes, urticaria, agranulocytosis, common with clozapine.

Interactive

1. Potentiates all CNS depressants hypnotics, anxiolytics, opioids, alcohol.
2. Block the actions of levodopa used for parkinsonism.
3. Abolish the antihypertensive effects of guanethidine, clonidine, methyldopa.

Uses

1. Psychosis
   - Schizophrenia
   - Mania
   - Anxiety (related to psychosis)
2. Antiemetic
   - Not used in morning sickness and motion sickness
3. Intractable hiccough (CPZ given I.V.).
4. Tetanus
   - CPZ is a secondary drug for muscle relaxation
5. Alcoholic hallucinosis, Huntington's disease.

Antidepressants

- Drugs which elevate mood.
- Affect monoaminergic transmission in the brain.
- Classification
1. Reversible inhibitors of MAO AI, clargyline, moclobemide
2. Tricyclic antidepressants (NA = Noradrenergic)
  A. NA + 5 HT uptake inhibitors,
     Imipramine, trimipramine, clemipramine, amitriptyline, doxepin, dothepin.
  B. NA uptake inhibitors: Desipramine, nortryptilline, amoxapin.
3. Selective serotonin reuptake inhibitors (SSRI)
   Fluroxetine, paroxetine, fluvoxamine, sertoline citacopram.
4. Atypical antidepressants: Trazodone, mianserin, mitazapine, venlafaxine, buproprien, tianeptine, amireptine.

TRICYCLE ANTIDEPRESSANTS (TCA)

Pharmacological Actions

Tricycle antidepressants (TCA's) inhibit monoamine reuptake and interacts with various receptors like mucuranic, histamine H_1, 5-HT, 5-HT_2 and dopamine.

1. CNS - In normal individuals' clumsiness, less concentrations and thinking, light headedness, sleepiness.

   In depressed individuals sedation appears first, after 2 to 3 weeks, mood is elevated, patients are communicative and start taking interest in surroundings.

TCA's lower the seizure threshold and cause convulsion in overdose clanipramine, maprotiline buproprien, and amoxthpine have highest seizure precipetating potential.

Mechanism of Action: Inhibits the uptake of NA and 5-HT into the respective neurons, and thus potentiate them.

TCA's may indirectly facilitate dopaminergic transmission in forebrain that may add to mood elevated action.

Uptake blockade occurs quickly, but anti-depressant action develops after weeks. Initially α_2 and $5HT_1$ receptors are activated, resulting in decreased firing at locus caseruleus (NA) and raphe (serotogenic). However, on long term, these receptors are desensitized. The end resultis increased amount of NA and 5HT, and thus transmission.

3. ANS: Anticholinergic action. Potentiate exogenous and endogenous NA, but have a blocking property as well.
4. CVS: Due to anticholinergic and NA potentiating effects, tachycardia, postural hypotension.

ECG: Interference with intraventricular conduction, T wave depression.

Tolerance and Dependence

To anticholinergic and hypotensive effects develop gradually.

Pharmacokinetics

Oral absorption is good, but slow. Bound to plasma tissue protein. Metabolized in liver their t½ is longer, so once daily dosing can be done.

Therapeutic Window: 50 to 200 µg/dL, optimal antidepressant effects are executed at a narrow band of plasma concentration.

Adverse Effects

i. Anticholinergic.
ii. Sedative, mental confusion.
iii. Increased, appetite and weight gain and with TCA's and trazodone.
iv. Sweating and tremors.
v. Seizure threshold is lowered.
vi. Cardiac arrhythmias.
vii. Rashes and jaundice due to hypersensitivity reactions.

Drug Interactions

1. TCA's potentiate sympathomimetic amines (cold/asthma) and inhibit indirect acting sympathi-comimetic (ephedrine, tyramine).
2. Abolish acute hypertensive effect of guane-thidine, clonidine α-methyldopa.
3. Potentiate CNS depressants.
4. Phenytoin, phenylbutazone, aspirin and CPZ displace TCA's from their protein binding site, causing toxicity.
5. Antiepileptics induce the metabolism of TCA's.
6. SSRI inhibit TCA metabolism, dangerous toxicity can occurs, if two are given together.
7. When used with anticholinergics, both actions may add up.
8. MAO inhibitors—Dangerous hypertensive crises may occur.

Selective Serotonin Re-uptake inhibitors (SSRIs)

They resemble TCAs in efficacy, but lack the side effects, caused by later, e.g., anticholinergic, cardio-vascular, neurological, and lag time of 2 to 4 weeks before the antidepressant action.

- No sedation, impairment of cognitive function.
- No beta adinergic blocking action.
- No seizures.

Side effects: Impairment of platelet function, tachymosis, epistaxis are frequent.
- Gastric blood loss due to NSAIDs.

Drug Interactions
- Inhibit metabolising isoenzymes, and thus elevate plasma levels of TCA, haloperidol, clozapine, warfarin, -blockers, benzodi-azepines.
- Drug interactions are least with sertaline and citalopram.

Atypical Antidepressants
1. Trazodone
   - Blocks 5-HT uptake.
   - Prominent b_1 blocking action causes bradycardia, priapism postural hypo-tension.
2. Mianserine
   - Block $beta_2$ receptors, increases NA turnover in brain.
   - It is sedative.
   - Blood dyscrasias and liver dysfunction is reported.
3. Tianeptine
   - It increases 5 HT uptake.
   - Used in anxio depressive states.
4. Amineptine
   - Enhances 5 HT uptake.
   - Has anticholinergic side effects.
5. Venlafaxine
   - Serotonin and NA reuptake inhibitor.
   - A noval antidepressant, has least side effects, preferred over TCAs.
6. Mirtazapine
   - Blocks $Beta_2$ and 5HT receptors, enhances NA and 5-HT release.
   - Augment NA, further increases firing of serotonergic raphe.
   - Labelled as (NaSSA) noradrenergic and specific serotonergic antidepressant.
7. Bupropion.
   - Inhibits DA and NA uptake.
   - Used as an aid in smoking cessation.
   - Seizure occur at higher doses.

MAO INHIBITORS[2]
- MAO is a mitochondrial enzyme which causes oxidative amination of biogenic amines (WA, DA, 5 HT, adrenaline).

(a) MAO-A—Deaminates 5 HT and NA.
(b) MAO-B—Deaminates phenyl ethylamine, and is inhibited by serigeline.
   Dopamine is degraded by both.
   MAO-A—Peripheral adrenergic nerve endings, intestinal mucosa, human placenta.
   MAO-B—Brain and platelets, liver contains both.

Interactions
(i) Cheese reaction
(ii) Enhances effects of levodopa, cold remedies, anticholinergics.

Reversible inhibitors of MAO
1. Maclobemide:
   - Lacks anticholinergic, sedative, cognitive and CVS side effects.
   - MAO activity is restored in 1-2 days.

Uses of Antidepressant Drugs
(i) Major depression.

(ii) Obsessive compulsive and phobic states.
(iii) Anxiety disorders (SSRIs especially in post traumatic stress disorders).
(iv) Neuropathic pain.
(v) Attention deficit—hyperactive disorder in children.
(vi) Enureis.
(vii) Migraine.
(viii) Pruritus.

Lithium
- Antimaniac/mood stabilizing drug.
- Used in bipolar maniac depressive illness.

Pharmacological Action
1. CNS: No acute effects, but on prolonged administration, it acts as a mood stabiliser (1 to 2 weeks). Sleep pattern is normalized.

Mechanism of Action
(a) Li^+ partly displaces Na^+ and is nearly equally distributed extracellularly as well as intracellularly.
(b) Li^+ decreases release of NA and DA in the brain.
(c) It inhibits inositol-1-P hydrolysis, thus IP_3 and DAG are not generated which is required for hyperactive neurone of the manic patients.
2. Inhibits ADH—increases urine output.
3. Has insulin like action on glucose metabolism.
4. Leucocyte count is increased by lithium therapy.
5. It decreases thyroxine synthesis by interference with coordination of tyrosine.

Pharmacokinetics
- Well absorbed orally.
- Neither protein neither bound nor metabolized.
- It is fully distributed extracellularly and then slowly penetrates into the CNS.
- The renal handling of Li^+ is much the same as Na^+, i.e., absorbed in proximal tubules.
  Li^+ is rapidly excreted after single bolus dose in 10–12 hours but thereafter, slowly reaches a steady plasma concentration in 5 to 7 days.
- Since margin of safety is low, measurement of serum Li concentration is measured every 12 hours after last dose.
  0.5 to 0.8 mEq/L–Bipolar illness
  0.8 to 1.1 mEq/L–Acute episodes
  > 1.5 mEq/L–Toxicity
  (more in elderly and patients of renal failure)
- It is excreted in saliva, breast milk and sweat.

Adverse Effects
(i) Nausea and vomiting
(ii) Thirst and polyuria.
(iii) CNS toxicity coarse tremors, giddiness, ataxia, motor incoordination, slurred speech, hyperreflexia, overdose symptoms occur > 2 mEq/L.
It progresses to delirium, convulsions and coma.

Treatment
- Symptomatic
  Osmotic diuresis
  Soda bicarbonate

(iv) Long term use:
   Diabetes insipidus
   Goitre
(v) Contraindicated in pregnancy
   - Foetal goitre
   - Also contraindicated in sick liver syndrome.

Interactions

(i) Diuresis (thiazide, fursemide) reabsorption of Na^+ as well as Li^+, toxicity can occur.
(ii) Tetracycline, ACE inhibitor cause Li^+ retention.
(iii) Enhances hypoglycaemia due to insulin.
(iv) Suxamethonium and pancuronium cause marked prolonged paralysis in Li^+ treated patients.

Uses

1. Acute manic episodes.
2. Prophylaxis in bipolar disorders.
3. Cancer chemotherapy induced leucopenia.

Tricyclic Antidepressants[2] (TCA)
- Continue dose before surgery.
- Requirement of drugs increases due to secretion of more neuro transmitter.
- Exaggerated BP response due to increase in NA.
- Indirect acting vasopressor like epidrine is avoided.
- Hypertensive crises occur in acute treatment (14-21 days).
- Cardiac A/V block.
  Treatment with atropine
- Chronic therapy: Pancuronium—Tachy arrhy-thmias.
- Enflurane—Seizure inducing potential.
- Adrenaline rinsed local anaesthesics all avoided—due to chances of hypertension.

MonoAmino oxidase Inhibitors (MAOIs)

Nonselective: (Phenelzine, isocarboxid, tranyl– cypromine) Anticholinergic, ketamine, pancuronium avoided, Suxamethonium inhibits pseudo cholinesterase. Postoperative analgesia: Opioids/fentanyl in small dose. Intraoperative: Sympathetic stimulation is prevented. Indirect acting vasopressor is used if hypotension occurs.

Lithium
- Avoid Diuretics
- Give Na^+ containing solutions as with hyponatremia, Li^+ will be reabsorbed.
- Give titrating dose of inhalational IV inducing agents so as to prevent sedation and myocardial depression due to Li^+
- ECG monitoring
- Duration of blockade by suxamethonium, NDMRs may be prolonged.

Antipsychotic
- $Beta_1$ blockade : Chances of hypotension and also compensatory mechanism fail.
- Predisposes to ventricular tachycardia (QT interval prolonged).
- Dose of IV and inhalational agents is decreased as prolonged sedation may occur.

References
1. Miller J. Anesthesia 6th Ed. Philadelphia, Churchill-Livingstone, 2004.
2. Kumar P. Textbook of Anaesthesia. Hyderabad, Paras Pub Med ,2007

Chapter 13.   Paediatric Drugs and Dosage

Acetaminophen
Analgesic and antipyretic.
  PO/PR: 40-60 mg/kg/day ÷ q4-6h (maximum 60 mg/kg or 4 g/day).
A single dose greater than 150 mg/kg is generally considered to be toxic, but toxicity has been reported at lower doses (90-120 mg/kg/day). Rectal absorption may be erratic, consider increasing dose by approximately 20%.
1 microgram/mL = 6.62 micromol/mL.

Weight (kg)	Single Dose (mg)
2.5 - 3.9	40
4.0 - 5.4	60
5.5 - 7.9	80
8.0 - 10.9	120
11.0 - 15.9	160
16.0 - 21.9	240
22.0 - 26.9	320
27.0 - 31.9	400
32.0 - 43.9	480
44 – over	650

Acetazolamide
Carbonic anhydrase inhibitor diuretic.
  Diuretic:
  PO: 5-10 mg/kg/day ÷ q8-24h (maximum 1 g/day).
Increases urinary bicarbonate loss and alkalinizes urine.

Acetylcysteine
  Antidote for acetaminophen overdose:
  IV: Total dose 300 mg/kg IV over 21 hours:
    150 mg/kg over 1 hour then
    50 mg/kg over 4 hours then
    100 mg/kg over 16 hours
Longer courses of therapy may be indicated if delayed presentation or slow resolution of liver function abnormalities. If symptoms of histamine release and brochospasm occur, hold infusion, give anti-histamines +/- corticosteroids and brochodilators, then restart infusion.

Acetylsalicylic Acid
  Antiplatelet:
  PO: 5 mg/kg/dose q24h.
    Minimum 20 mg, usual maximum 80 or 325 mg.
  Kawasaki disease:
  PO: 80-100 mg/kg/day ÷ q6h, reduce dose to 3-5 mg/kg q24h once fever resolves.
Supplied as 80 mg chewable tablets and 325 and 650 mg tablets.

Activated Charcoal
  see Charcoal

Acyclovir
Antiviral.
  Herpes simplex encephalitis:
  IV: 45 mg/kg/day ÷ q8h (60 mg/kg/day has been used in infants).
  Other herpes simplex infections:
  IV: 15-30 mg/kg/day ÷ q8h.
  Varicella (severe) or in immunocompromised hosts:
  IV: 30-45 mg/kg/day ÷ q8h, switch to PO when lesions crusted.
  PO: 80 mg/kg/day ÷ qid (maximum 800 mg/dose).
Ensure adequate urine output. Adjust dosing interval in renal impairment.

Adenosine
Antiarrhythmic.
Treatment of SVT:
IV: 0.1 mg/kg bolus (maximum 6 mg),
if no response in 2 min: 0.2 mg/kg bolus (maximum 12 mg).
Not effective for atrial fibrillation/flutter or ventricular fibrillation. Adverse effects such as dyspnea, arrhythmias, bradycardia, flushing, sinus and AV block are very common but are usually transient due to short (10 seconds) half-life of drug. Give rapid IV bolus followed by rapid NS flush.

Albumin
Colloid plasma volume expander (human plasma protein).
IV: 0.5-1 g/kg/dose:
5% solution (50 mg/mL): 10-20 mL/kg/dose.
25% solution (250 mg/mL): 2-4 mL/kg/dose.
Use 5% solution for fluid resuscitation and volume expansion, 25% albumin is very viscous and hyperosmolar, use with caution.

Alprostadil
Prostoglandin E_1.
Maintenance of patent ductus arteriosus:
IV: Initially 0.05 microgram/kg/min, use lowest effective dose, 0.01-0.1 microgram/kg/min has been used.

May cause apnea, be prepared to intubate. Most effective in infants less than 96 hours of age.

Alteplase
Thrombolytic.
Unblocking of occluded catheters:
Intracatheter: Instill 1 mg/mL solution into occluded lumen. Maximum volume equal to the internal volume of catheter lumen, to maximum of 2 mL. Leave in place for 30 min-2h, then **aspirate solution. Do not infuse.** May repeat once if ineffective.

Amikacin
Neonatal Dosing

Dosing Table for IV Systemic Administration			
PMA (wk)	Postnatal (d)	Dose (mg/kg)	Interval (h)
≤29	0-7	18	48
	8-28	15	36
	≥29	15	24
30-34	0-7	18	36
	≥8	15	24
≥35	All	15	24

Abbreviation: PMA, postmenstrual age.

Infant, Children, and Adolescent Dosing
CONVENTIONAL DOSING: 5 to 7.5 mg/kg/dose every 8 hours
DOSAGE FOR RENAL IMPAIRMENT: Yes

Monitoring in neonates
WHEN TO DRAW LEVELS
- Peak: After second dose (see "Timing of Levels").
- Trough: After second dose (just before third dose).
- Levels are unnecessary if patient is on antibiotics for 48 to 72 hour rule-out sepsis protocol.
- Consider more frequent monitoring in hypothermia treatment.

TIMING OF LEVELS
- Peak: 30 minutes after end of 30-minute infusion
- Trough: 0 to 30 minutes before next dose

GOAL LEVELS
- Amikacin peak: 20 to 25 mcg/mL.
- Amikacin trough: <5 mcg/mL.

Amikacin
Aminoglycoside antibiotic.
   IV: 15-20 mg/kg/day ÷ q12-24h.
Adjust dosing interval in renal impairment. Ototoxicity and nephrotoxicity may occur, consider monitoring trough levels (<5-10 mg/L) in patients at risk for nephrotoxicity; septic shock, concurrent nephrotoxins, fluctuating renal function or extended treatment courses. May potentiate muscle weakness with neuromuscular blockers. Reserved for gram negative organisms with documented resistance to other aminoglycosides.

Aminocaproic Acid
Fibrinolysis inhibitor.
   <u>Treatment of excessive bleeding due to hyperfibrinolysis:</u>
   IV: 50-100 mg/kg then 30-50 mg/kg/h until bleeding stops
         (maximum 1 g/h).
Rapid IV injection may cause hypotension, bradycardia, arrhythmias. Give loading dose over 1 hour.

Aminophylline
Xanthine derivative used to treat reversible airway obstruction.
   <u>Acute bronchospasm:</u>
   IV: 6 mg/kg then infusion (based on ideal body weight):
         2-6 months: 0.4-0.5 mg/kg/h
         6-11 months: 0.6-0.7 mg/kg/h
         1-12 years: 0.8-1 mg/kg/h
         >12 years   0.7 mg/kg/h
No longer first line for treatment of asthma, high dose inhaled/IV β_2 agonists and corticosteroids are preferred. Dose adjustments are required in CHF, liver dysfunction, multisystem organ failure, shock and in smokers. Drug interactions are common, including ciprofloxacin, clarithromycin, erythromycin. Draw level 30 minutes after end of bolus infusion and 12-24 hours after initiation of continuous infusion.
Target serum level is 10-15 mg/L (55-83 micromol/mL).

Amiodarone
Antiarrhythmic.
   IV: 5 mg/kg loading dose then 5-15 microgram/kg/min.
Give loading dose over 20-60 minutes for perfusing rhythms or rapid bolus for VF. Rapid IV boluses are limited to the treatment of VF because of the associated hypotension, which may respond to reducing the infusion rate. Heart block requiring pacing has occurred. Do not use in cardiogenic shock, severe sinus node dysfunction, sinus bradycardia, 2nd and 3rd degree AV block. Central line required for concentrations >2 mg/mL.

Amlodipine
Calcium channel blocker antihypertensive.
   PO: 0.1-0.3 mg/kg q24h (usual maximum 10 mg/day).

Amoxicillin
Penicillin derivative oral antibiotic.
   PO: 25-50 mg/kg/day ÷ q8h (maximum 1 g/dose).
For severe infections and for suspected penicillin resistant S. pneumoniae doses of up to 100 mg/kg/day have been tolerated (maximum 1 g/dose). Use ampicillin if IV therapy is required.

Amoxicillin/Clavulanic Acid
Penicillin derivative antibiotic and beta-lactamase inhibitor.
   PO: 25-40 mg/kg/day of amoxicillin component ÷ q8h
         (maximum 500 mg/dose).
Active against gram positive, gram negative and anerobic organisms.

Amphotericin B (Amphotericin B Deoxycholate)
Antifungal.
- IV: 0.6-1 mg/kg/dose q24h (maximum 70 mg/dose).

For Candida use 0.6-0.8 mg/kg/day and 1 mg/kg/day for Aspergillus. Traditionally give ½ dose on first day and increase to full dose over 1-2 days, but may give full dose on first day. Consider hydration (10 mL/kg of normal saline) pre-amphotericin to reduce the risk of nephrotoxicity. Commonly causes nephrotoxicity, hypokalemia and hypomagnesemia. Not compatible with any saline solutions, dilute to 0.1 mg/mL or less in dextrose solutions and infuse over 2-6 hours.

Amphotericin B Lipid Complex (Abelcet®) and Liposomal Amphotericin B (AmBisome®)
Antifungal (lipid formulations of amphotericin B).
- IV: 3-5 mg/kg q24h.

Consider using these in renal insufficiency, if nephrotoxicity develops while on standard Amphotericin B or with clinical failure with alternate agents. These lipid formulations are better tolerated but are very costly.

Ampicillin
Penicillin derivative antibiotic.

Meningitis:
- IV: 200 mg/kg/day ÷ q6h (maximum 2 g/dose).

Other infections:
- IV: 100-200 mg/kg/day ÷ q6h (maximum 2 g/dose).

Doses of 400 mg/kg/day have been used for meningitis. Adjust dosing interval in renal impairment. Use amoxicillin if oral therapy is required.

Arginine
Treatment of urea cycle disoders.

OTC or CPS deficiency:
- IV: 0.2 g/kg as a loading dose, then 0.2 g/kg/day as a continuous infusion.

ASL or ASS deficiency:
- IV: 0.6 g/kg as a loading dose, then 0.6 g/kg/day as a continuous infusion.

ASA/Aspirin
See acetylsalicylic acid.

Atracurium
Non-depolarizing neuromuscular blocking agent.
- IV: 0.4 mg/kg q30min prn

  or

  0.4 mg/kg then 2-15 microgram/kg/min.

Bolus dosing preferred. Does not require dosage modification in renal or hepatic impairment. Regular sedation, analgesia and ocular lubrication required. Monitor depth of paralysis using peripheral nerve stimulation when using infusions (target 1-2 twitches out of 4). Onset of action is within 2 minutes, duration of action is 30-40 minutes. Prolonged weakness may occur, especially when corticosteroids are used concurrently with non-depolarizing neuromuscular blocking agents.

Atropine
Vagolytic.

Bradycardia:
- IV: 0.02 mg/kg/dose, minimum dose: 0.1 mg,

  maximum dose: 0.5 mg for child, 1 mg for adolescent.

If giving via ETT, increase IV dose 2-10 fold and dilute to 3-5 mL with NS. Follow with several positive pressure breaths.

Azithromycin
Azolide antibiotic (related to the macrolides).
 PO/IV: 10 mg/kg (maximum 500 mg) once, then
    5 mg/kg (maximum 250 mg) q24h x 4.
    For serious infections may give 10 mg/kg q24h.
  <u>Chlamydial infection (non-gonococcal urethritis or cervicitis):</u>
 PO: 1 g once (minimum weight 45 kg).

Budesonide
Inhaled corticosteroid.
 NEB: 0.25-1 mg bid via nebulizer.

Calcium
Electrolyte.
 Treatment of hypocalcemia, hyperkalemia, hypermagnesemia and calcium channel antagonist overdose. These doses are suggested starting doses, increase and repeat as required.
<u>Calcium Gluconate:</u>
 IV: 50-100 mg of calcium gluconate/kg/dose (0.5-1 mL/kg/dose)
  or
 IV: Add 1 g of calcium gluconate to a total of 50 mL NS (0.046 mmol/mL) and give 0.05-0.1 mmol/kg/h (1-2 mL/kg/h), adjust rate q4h.

<u>Calcium Chloride:</u>
 IV: 10-20 mg of calcium chloride/kg/dose (0.1-0.2 mL/kg/dose).

	Elemental Calcium		
Calcium gluconate 10% (100 mg/mL)	9 mg/mL	0.45 mEq/mL	0.23 mmol/mL
Calcium chloride 10% (100 mg/mL)	27.2 mg/mL	1.4 mEq/mL	0.7 mmol/mL

If treating asymptomatic hypocalcemia infuse dose over at least 1 hour.

Captopril
Angiotensin converting enzyme inhibitor.
 PO: 0.1-0.3 mg/kg/dose q8h initially
   (usual maximum 6 mg/kg/day or 200 mg/day).
Monitor blood pressure closely after first dose, may cause profound hypotension.

Carbamazepine
Anticonvulsant.
 PO: 10-20 mg/kg/day initially, usual maintenance dose is
   20-30 mg/kg/day. Divide daily dose q8-12h.
Serum trough concentration target is 17-51 micromol/L (4-12 microgram/mL).

Cefaclor
Oral second generation cephalosporin.
 PO: 20-40 mg/kg/day ÷ q8h (maximum 1.5 g/day).
Adjust dosing interval in renal impairment. Do not give with food.
Non-formulary at Hamilton Health Sciences.

Cefazolin
First generation cephalosporin.
 IV: 75-150 mg/kg/day ÷ q8h (maximum 6 g/day).
Adjust dosing interval in renal impairment.

Cefixime
Oral third generation cephalosporin.
 PO: 8 mg/kg/day ÷ q12-24h (maximum 400 mg/day).
  <u>Uncomplicated cervical/urethral gonorrhea:</u>
 PO: 400 mg once (minimum weight 45 kg).
Adjust dose in renal impairment. Not active against Pseudomonas aeruginosa or Staphlococcus aureus. Restricted at Hamilton Health Sciences to the treatment of STDs.

Cefotaxime
Third generation cephalosporin.
> Meningitis:
> IV: 200 mg/kg/day ÷ q6h (maximum 8 g/day).
> Other infections:
> IV: 100-200 mg/kg/day ÷ q8h (maximum 6 g/day).

Adjust dosing interval in renal impairment. Not active against Pseudomonas aeruginosa.

Cefotetan
Second generation cephalosporin.
> IV: 60 mg/kg/day ÷ q12h (maximum 6 g/day).

Adjust dosing interval in renal impairment. Active against anerobic organisms. Non-formulary at Hamilton Health Sciences.

Cefoxitin
Second generation cephalosporin.
> IV: 80-160 mg/kg/day ÷ q8h (maximum 8 g/day).

Adjust dosing interval in renal impairment. Active against anerobic organisms. Non-formulary at Hamilton Health Sciences.

Cefprozil
Oral second generation cephalosporin.
> PO: 30 mg/kg/day ÷ q12h (maximum 1 g/day).

Adjust dose in severe renal impairment.

Ceftazidime
Third generation cephalosporin.
> IV: 75-150 mg/kg/day ÷ q8h (maximum 6 g/day).

Adjust dosing interval in renal impairment. Active against Pseudomonas aeruginosa.

Ceftriaxone
Third generation cephalosporin.
> Meningitis:
> IV/IM: 80 mg/kg/dose q12 hours x 3 doses then q24h (maximum 2 g/dose).
> Other infections:
> IV/IM: 50-75 mg/kg q24h (maximum 2 g/day).

No dosage adjustment required in renal impairment. Not active against Pseudomonas aeruginosa. Restricted at Hamilton Health Sciences to patients without IV access, otherwise use cefotaxime.

Cefuroxime/Cefuroxime Axetil
Second generation cephalosporin.
> Epiglottitis/facial cellulitis:
> IV: 150 mg/kg/day ÷ q8h (maximum 1.5 g/dose)
> Other infections:
> IV: 75-150 mg/kg/day ÷ q8h (usual maximum dose is 750 mg/dose)
> PO: 20-30 mg/kg/day ÷ bid (maximum 1 g/day)

Adjust dosing interval in renal impairment. Oral formulation is non-formulary at Hamilton Health Sciences.

Cephalexin
First generation cephalosporin.
> PO: 25-50 mg/kg/day ÷ qid, for severe infections can give 100 mg/kg/day (maximum 4 g/day).

Adjust dosing interval in renal impairment.

Charcoal
Adsorbent used in toxic ingestions.
> PO: 1-2 g/kg once.
> PO: Multiple dose therapy 0.5 g/kg q4-6h.

Give via NG if necessary, consider antiemetics.

Chloral Hydrate
Sedative and hypnotic.
> Procedural Sedation:
> PO/PR: 80 mg/kg, may repeat half dose if no effect in 30 minutes (maximum 2 g/dose).
> Sedation:
> PO/PR: 25-50 mg/kg/dose (maximum 500 mg q6h or 1 g hs).

Avoid in liver dysfunction. Tolerance develops and withdrawal may occur after long-term use. For PR use dilute syrup with water.

Ciprofloxacin
Quinolone antibiotic.
> IV/PO: 20-30 mg/kg/day ÷ q12h
> (maximum 400 mg/dose IV or 750 mg/dose PO).

Excellent oral absorption, use IV only if PO contraindicated. Feeds, formula, calcium, magnesium, iron, antacids and sulcralfate reduce absorption, hold feeds for 1 hour before and 2 hours after dose. Adjust dosing interval in renal impairment. Ciprofloxacin has been used in pediatrics but the association between ciprofloxacin and the development of arthropathy in humans is still controversial. Active against Pseudomonas aeruginosa.

Cloxacillin
Beta-lactamase-resistant penicillin.
> IV: 100-200 mg/kg/day ÷ q6h (maximum 8 g/day).
> PO: 25-50 mg/kg/day ÷ q6h (maximum 500 mg/dose).

Higher oral doses are poorly tolerated, usually use cephalexin instead. Primarily used in Staphylococcal infections.

Codeine
Opiate analgesic used to treat mild-moderate pain.
> PO/IM/SC: 0.5-1 mg/kg q4h prn (maximum 60 mg/dose).

Not for IV use due to significant histamine release and possible cardiovascular side effects. Not commonly used in ICU setting.

Co-trimoxazole (Trimethoprim/Sulfamethoxazole)
Sulfa derivative antibiotic.
> Bacterial infections:
> PO/IV: 8 mg/kg/day (of trimethoprim component) ÷ q12h.
> Pneumocystis carinii pneumonia (PCP):
> PO/IV: 20 mg/kg/day (of trimethoprim component) ÷ q6h.

Excellent oral absorption, use IV only if PO contraindicated. Maintain good fluid intake and urine output. Adjust dosing interval in renal impairment. Monitor CBC and LFTs. Do not use in patients with G-6-PD deficiency. If PCP is severe (i.e. hypoxia), consider adding methylprednisolone 1 mg/kg q24h.

Order in mL of suspension or injection or number of tablets:
> Suspension: 8 mg trimethoprim and 40 mg sulfamethoxazole/mL.
> Injection: 16 mg trimethoprim and 80 mg sulfamethoxazole/mL.
> Tablet: 80 mg trimethoprim and 400 mg sulfamethoxazole.
> DS tablet: 160 mg trimethoprim and 800 mg sulfamethoxazole.

Cisatracurium
Non-depolarizing neuromuscular blocking agent.
- IV: 0.1 mg/kg then 0.03 mg/kg prn
  or
  0.1 mg/kg then 1-3 microgram/kg/min
  (range 0.5-10 microgram/kg/min).

Bolus dosing preferred. Does not require dosage modification in renal or hepatic impairment. Regular sedation, analgesia and ocular lubrication required. Monitor depth of paralysis using peripheral nerve stimulation when using infusions (target 1-2 twitches out of 4). Onset of action within 2-3 minutes, duration of action is 30-40 minutes. Prolonged weakness may occur, especially when corticosteroids are used concurrently with non-depolarizing neuromuscular blocking agents

Clarithromycin
Macrolide antibiotic.
- PO: 15 mg/kg/day ÷ q12h (maximum 1 g/day).

Drug interactions include theophylline, carbamazepine, cisapride, digoxin, cyclosporine, tacrolimus. Adjust dose in severe renal impairment.

Clindamycin
Antibiotic.
- IV: 30-40 mg/kg/day ÷ q8h (maximum 900 mg/dose).
- PO: 10-20 mg/kg/day ÷ q6-8h (maximum 450 mg/dose).

May potentate muscle weakness with neuromuscular blockers. Oral suspension is very poorly tolerated, avoid if possible, use 150 mg capsules or an alternative antibiotic. Active against gram positive and anaerobic organisms.

Cyclosporine
Immunosuppressant.
IV dose is approximately 50% of oral dose. Dose and serum levels vary widely with indication and the individual protocol, but usually:
- IV: 3-6 mg/kg/day ÷ q12h.
- PO: 5-10 mg/kg/day ÷ q12h.

Requires dose reduction in liver or renal dysfunction. Cyclosporine interacts with many medications, including fluconazole, erythromycin, tacrolimus, diltiazem, methylprednisolone, grapefruit juice, phenytoin, phenobarbital, carbamazepine, trimethoprim. Trough levels usually 100-300 microgram/L but varies with the indication.

Desmopressin (DDAVP)
Analogue of vasopressin.

Diabetes Insipidus:
- Nasal: 2.5-10 microgram/dose q12-24h.
- IV/IM/SC: 0.25-1 microgram/dose q12-24h
  (maximum 4 microgram/dose).

Coagulopathy:
- IV/SC: 0.3 microgram/kg/dose
  (maximum 20 microgram/dose).

Used as replacement therapy in diabetes insipidus, treatment of prolonged bleeding times and mild bleeding associated with some types of hemophilia. Parenteral dose is approximately 10% of intranasal dose and 1% of the oral dose. In the treatment of diabetes insipidus check urine output, volume status, serum and urine electrolytes prior to each dose.
Nasal spray=10 microgram/puff, nasal solution = 100 microgram/mL.

Dexamethasone
Corticosteroid.
> Croup:
> IV/IM/PO: 0.6 mg/kg once.
> Meningitis:
> IV: 0.15 mg/kg/dose q6h for 4 days.
>   Begin with first antibiotic dose.
> Prevention of post-extubation stridor:
> IV: 0.25-0.5 mg/kg/dose (maximum 10 mg/dose) q6h x 6 doses.
>   Begin 24 hours pre-extubation if possible.
> Increased ICP due to space occupying lesion:
> IV/PO: 0.2-0.4 mg/kg initially followed by
>   0.3 mg/kg/day ÷ q6h.

Discontinuation of therapy >14 days requires gradual tapering. Consider supplemental steroids at times of stress if patient has received long-term or frequent bursts of steroid therapy. Prolonged weakness may occur when corticosteroids are used concurrently with non-depolarizing neuromuscular blocking agents.

Dextrose
> Treatment of hypoglycemia:
> IV: 0.5-1 g/kg/dose:
>   1-2 mL/kg of 50% dextrose
>   5-10 mL/kg of 10% dextrose

1 mmol of dextrose (0.2 g of dextrose) provides 2.8 kJ (0.67 kcal).

Diazepam
Benzodiazepine sedative, anxiolytic and amnestic.
> Status epilepticus:
> IV: 0.25 mg/kg/dose (maximum 5 mg, 10 mg for older children).
> PR: 0.5 mg/kg/dose (maximum 20 mg/dose).
> ICU sedation:
> IV: 0.1-0.3 mg/kg q1h prn.

Fast onset and short duration of action with single doses, duration of action prolonged with continued use. Not first line drug for ICU sedation due to short duration of action and the potential for accumulation. Withdrawal may occur if discontinued abruptly after prolonged use. Not recommended for continuous infusion due to poor solubility. Can give parenteral preparation rectally, diluted with water.

Digoxin

	Total Digitalization Dose (maximum 1 mg) **Divide dose** q6h x 3 doses.		Maintenance Dose (usual maximum 250 mcg/day) Begin 12 h after last loading dose.	
	PO	IV	PO	IV
37 weeks-2 y	50 mcg/kg	35 mcg/kg	10 mcg/kg/day	8 mcg/kg/day
> 2 years	40 mcg/kg	30 mcg/kg	8 mcg/kg/day	6 mcg/kg/day

Usually divide daily maintenance dose q12h if less than 10 years of age, otherwise give dose once daily. Doses based on ideal body weight, decrease dose for patients with renal impairment. Digoxin has many drug interactions including nifedipine, verapamil, amiodarone, erythromycin, cisapride and sucralfate. IV dose is approximately 80% of PO dose. Monitor trough levels (0.5-2 microgram/L or 1-2.6 micromol/L).

Dimenhydrinate
Antihistamine used to treat nausea and vomiting.
> IV/IM/PO: 1 mg/kg/dose q4-6h (maximum 50 mg/dose).

Diphenhydramine
Antihistamine used primarily to treat urticaria.
    IV/IM/PO: 0.5-1 mg/kg/dose q6h (maximum 50 mg/dose).

Divalproex
    See valproic acid.

Dobutamine
Inotrope.
    IV: 2-20 microgram/kg/min.
Correct hypovolemia first to prevent hypotension. Give via central line if possible.

Domperidone
Prokinetic agent.
    PO: 1.2-2.4 mg/kg/day ÷ q6h (maximum 80 mg/day).

Dopamine
Vasopressor and inotrope.
    Hypotension and shock:
    IV: 2-20 microgram/kg/min.
Correct hypovolemia first. Consider changing to, or adding another drug at 15-20 microgram/kg/min or if tachycardia occurs. Give via central line if possible.

Drotecogin Alfa (Activated)
Recombinant human activated protein C.
    Severe sepsis:
    IV: 24 microgram/kg/h for 96h.
Anticoagulant and anti-inflammatory. There is limited experience with the use of drotecogin in pediatrics.

Epinephrine (Racemic)
    Post-extubation stridor/croup:
    NEB: 0.25-0.5 mL of 2.25% solution via nebulizer prn

Erythromycin
Macrolide antibiotic.
    IV: 25-50 mg/kg/day ÷ q6h (maximum 4 g/day).
    PO: 20-40 mg/kg/day ÷ q6h (maximum 2 g/day).
Has many drug interactions, may increase levels of midazolam, carbamazepine, theophylline, cyclosporine, phenytoin. GI adverse effects common, even with IV use. Thrombophlebitis common.

Esmolol
Short acting β blocking agent.
    Atrial fibrillation/atrial flutter/SVT/hypertension:
    IV: 100-500 microgram/kg then 50-300 microgram/kg/min.
        Titrate by 50-100 microgram/kg/min q5-10min.
        High doses of 500-1000 micrograms/kg/min have been rarely required.
Short-term use only, consider bolus dose with each increase in infusion. Change to longer acting agent once desired effect achieved. Duration of action is approximately 10 minutes.

Ethacrynic Acid
Loop diuretic.
    IV: 0.5-1 mg/kg/dose.
Use only if poor response to appropriate doses of furosemide. Repeat doses are not usually recommended but has been given q8-12h.

Enalapril or Enalaprilat
Angiotensin converting enzyme inhibitor.
> Hypertension, CHF:
> PO: 0.1 mg/kg/day ÷ q12-24h, increase as required
> (maximum 0.5 mg/kg/day or 40 mg/day).
> IV: 5-10 microgram/kg/dose q6-12h, titrated to clinical effect (usual maximum 30 microgram/kg/dose or 5 mg/dose).

Monitor blood pressure closely. There is limited experience with the use of IV enalaprilat in pediatrics. Enalaprilat is the IV formulation of enalpril.

Enoxaparin
Anticoagulant, low-molecular weight heparin.
> Treatment:
> SC: <2 months of age: 1.5 mg/kg/dose q12h.
> >2 months of age: 1 mg/kg/dose q12h.
> Prophylaxis:
> SC: <2 months of age: 0.75 mg/kg/dose q12h.
> >2 months of age: 0.5 mg/kg/dose q12h.

Monitor platelets and hemoglobin. Avoid in severe renal dysfunction. Anti-factor Xa level drawn 4 hours post SC injection should be 0.5-1 unit/mL for treatment and 0.2-0.4 unit/mL for prophylaxis.

Epinephrine
Vasopressor and inotrope.
> Symptomatic bradycardia or pulseless arrest:
> IV: 0.01 mg/kg/dose (0.1 mL/kg of 1:10 000 solution).
> ETT: 0.1 mg/kg/dose (0.1 mL/kg of 1:1000 solution).
> Refractory hypotension/shock:
> IV: 0.1-1 microgram/kg/min
> (doses of 0.01-1 microgram/kg/min have been used).
> Post-extubation stridor/croup:
> NEB: 2.5-5 mg/dose (2.5-5 mL of 1:1000 solution) prn.

1:10 000 solution = 0.1 mg/mL and 1:1 000 solution = 1 mg/mL.

Gentamicin

Neonatal Dosing

Dosing Table for IV Systemic Administration			
PMA (wk)	Postnatal (d)	Dose (mg/kg)	Interval (h)
<29	0-7	5	48
	8-28	4	36
	>29	4	24
30-34	0-7	4.5	36
	>8	4	24
>35	All	4	24

Abbreviation: PMA, postmenstrual age

Infant, Children, and Adolescent Dosing

CONVENTIONAL DOSING:
- Infants and children younger than 5 years: 2.5 mg/kg/dose every 8 hours
- Children 5 years and older: 2 to 2.5 mg/kg/dose every 8 hours

HIGH-DOSE, EXTENDED INTERVAL DOSING (IN PATIENTS WITH NORMAL RENAL FUNCTION): 5 to 7.5 mg/kg/dose every 24 hours

DOSAGE FOR RENAL IMPAIRMENT: Yes

Monitoring in Neonates

WHEN TO DRAW LEVELS
- Peak: After second dose (see "Timing of Levels").
- Trough: After second dose (just before third dose).
- Levels are unnecessary if patient is on antibiotics for 48 to 72 hour rule-out sepsis protocol.
- Consider more frequent monitoring in hypothermia treatment.

TIMING OF LEVELS
- Peak: 30 minutes after end of 30-minute infusion
- Trough: 0 to 30 minutes before next dose

Tobramycin

Neonatal Dosing

Dosing Table for IV Systemic Administration			
PMA (wk)	Postnatal (d)	Dose (mg/kg)	Interval (h)
≤29	0–7	5	48
	8–28	4	36
	≥29	4	24
30–34	0–7	4.5	36
	≥8	4	24
≥35	All	4	24

Abbreviation: PMA, postmenstrual age.

Infant, Children, and Adolescent Dosing

CONVENTIONAL DOSING:
- Infants and children younger than 5 years: 2.5 mg/kg/dose every 8 hours
- Children 5 years and older: 2 to 2.5 mg/kg/dose every 8 hours

CYSTIC FIBROSIS DOSING:
- Conventional CF dosing: 3.3 mg/kg/dose every 8 hours
- High-dose, extended interval dosing: 7 mg/kg/dose every 12 hours or 10 mg/kg/dose every 24 hours

DOSAGE FOR RENAL IMPAIRMENT: Yes

Monitoring in Neonates

WHEN TO DRAW LEVELS
- Peak: After second dose (see "Timing of Levels").
- Trough: After second dose (just before third dose).
- Levels are unnecessary if patient is on antibiotics for 48 to 72 hour rule-out sepsis protocol.

TIMING OF LEVELS
- Peak: 30 minutes after end of 30-minute infusion
- Trough: 0 to 30 minutes before next dose

GOAL LEVELS
- Tobramycin peak: 6 to 12 mcg/mL. (3 to 5 mcg/mL is an acceptable range for gram-positive synergy)
- Tobramycin trough: <1 mcg/mL

Monitoring in Infants, Children, and Adolescents

WHEN TO DRAW LEVELS
- Peak: After third dose (see "Timing of Levels").
- Trough: Prior third dose.
- Levels may be unnecessary if patient is on antibiotics for 48 to 72 hour rule-out sepsis protocol.

TIMING OF LEVELS
- Peak: 30 minutes after end of 30-minute infusion
- Trough: 0 to 30 minutes before next dose

GOAL LEVELS
- Tobramycin peak (non–cystic fibrosis dosing): 6 to 12 mcg/mL. (3 to 5 mcg/mL is an acceptable range for gram-positive synergy)
- Tobramycin peak (cystic fibrosis dosing): 8 to 14 mcg/mL
- Tobramycin trough: <2 mcg/mL. (<1 mcg/mL is ideal)

Vancomycin

Neonatal Dosing
Meningitis: 15 mg/kg/dose
Bacteremia: 10 mg/kg/dose

Dosing Table for IV Administration		
PMA (wk)	Postnatal (d)	Interval (h)
<29	0–14	18
	>14	12
30–36	0–14	12
	>14	8
37–44	0–7	12
	>7	8

Abbreviation: PMA, postmenstrual age

Infants, Children, and Adolescent Dosing

CONVENTIONAL DOSING: 15 to 20 mg/kg/dose every 6 to 8 hours (Consider every 6 hours for patients older than 2 months who do not have a history of cardial abnormalities.)

DOSAGE FOR RENAL IMPAIRMENT: Yes

Monitoring in Neonates
TROUGHS ONLY EXCEPT WITH
- Central nervous system infections
- Osteomyelitis
- Infective abscess
- Goal trough >10 mcg/ml

Monitoring in Infants, Children, and Adolescents
Only trough levels are recommended.

WHEN TO DRAW LEVELS
- Trough: Before third dose (for neonates) or fourth dose (for infants, children, and adolescents)
- Peak: After third dose (when necessary)

References
1. Miller J. Anesthesia 6th Ed. Philadelphia, Churchill-Livingstone, 2004.
2. Kumar P. Textbook of Anaesthesia. Hyderabad, Paras Pub Med ,2007
3. Pramod Kumar.Textbook of anaesthesia and analgesia. Part 1: Basic sciences. Ist Edn, Amazon Kindle, New York,2018

Chapter 14. Summary of drugs used in Anaesthesia

Table 1 - Drugs used in bronchial asthma

	Beta 2 agonists	Methylxanthines	Mast cell stabilizers	Corticosteroids
Drugs	Salbutamol, terbutaline, salmeterol	Theophylline, aminophylline, deriphylline	Sodium cromoglycate	Beclomethasone, budesonide, prednisolone
Mechanism of action	Stimulation of Beta 2 receptors	Release of calcium from sarcoplasmic reticulum, inhibit phosphodiesterase, block adenosine receptors	Inhibit degranulation of mast cells	Act on glucocorticoid receptor & Reduce bronchial hyperactivity, mucosal oedema, antiinflammatory
Dose	inhalation Salbutamol 100-200µg, terbutaline 250 µg, salmeterol-100-200 µg oral Salbutamol 2-4 mg, terbutaline-5mg	Theophylline – 15mg/kg/day oral Aminophylline-5mg/kg i.v	1 mg per dose, 2 puffs 4 times a day	Beclomethasone 50 µg bd inhalation, Prednisolone 20-40mg daily
Metabolism	Presystemic metabolism in gut	In liver	Unchanged in urine	In liver
Actions	Bronchodilation occurs in 10 min & lasts upto 6 hours, tachycardia,	CNS stimulation, tachycardia, smooth muscle relaxation, mild diuretics, inhibit histamine release	Anti-inflammatory	↑ gluconeogenesis, glycogen synthesis' ↓ inflammation, ↑ ICP
Uses	Mild to moderately severe cases	Asthma, COPD, apnoea in premature infants	Asthma, allergic rhinitis, allergic conjunctivitis	Severe chronic asthma, status asthmaticus
Side effects	Muscle tremors, palpitations, nervousness, ankle oedema	Dose related-nervousness, tremors, vomiting, palpitation, tachypnoea, extrasystoles, convulsions	Bronchospasm, throat irritation, cough, rashes	Cushing's habitus, purple stria, hyperglycemia, delayed healing, osteoporosis, suppression of hypothalamus

Also ipratrpium bromide is used in inhalation form for bronchodialtation in COPD patient, 2 puffs 20μg/puff 3-4 times daily

Table 2. Drugs of cardiovascular system

	Quinidine	Amiodarone	Verapamil	Nifedipine	diltiazem	Enalapril
Group	Antiarrhythmic	Antiarrhythmic	Calcium channel blocker	Calcium channel blocker	Calcium channel blocker	ACE inhibitor
Mechanism of action	Na+ channel blocker leading to membrane stabilization	Blocks potassium, calcium channels	• calcium mediated depolarization	• calcium mediated depolarization	• calcium mediated depolarization	ACE inhibitor
Dose	200-400mg tds oral	5mg/kg i.v over 30-60 min	40 -120 mg tds oral, 5-10 mg slow i.v	5-20mg bd oral, 10mg capsule bitten & swallowed every ½ to 1 hour	30 – 60 mg tds-qds	5-20 mg od-bd
Metabolism	In liver	In liver	In liver	In liver	In liver	In liver
Actions	• automaticity, • ERP in heart, • BP, irritant to GIT	• automaticity, • ERP, APD	• SA node automaticity, • ERP of AV node, vascular smooth muscle relaxation	Arteriolar dilatation, • BP, • heart rate	• SA node automaticity, Arteriolar dilatation	• BP, no fall in renal, coronary, cerebral blood flow
Uses	Atrial flutter, atrial fibrillation, ventricular extrasystole	Ventricular tachycardia, recurrent Ventricular fibrillation, supraventricular arrhythmias	PSVT, control ventricular rate in atrial flutter & atrial fibrillation, in angina patients	In hypertension, safe in pregnancy	Hypertension, angina, PSVT	Hypertension, diabetes nephropathy, CHF, MI, scleroderma crisis
Side effects	Gastrointestinal intolerance, hypersensitivity, torsades de pointes	Gastrointestinal intolerance, photosenitization, pulmonary alveolitis, peripheral neuropathy	Nausea, constipation, bradycardia, headache	Palpitation, flushing, ankle oedema, hypotension, headache, nausea	Nausea, constipation, bradycardia, headache	Hypotension, hyperkalemia, cough, fetal damage, headace, granulocytopenia

TABLE 3. Drugs used for hyperthyroid patient

Characteristics	Propythiouracil	Carbimazole	Methimazole	Iodides	Radioactive iodine
Group	Thioamide	Thioamide	Thioamide		
Mechanism if action	Inhibit iodination of tyrosine residues in thyroglobulin. Inhibit coupling of iodotyrosine residues to form T_3 and T_4. Inhibits conversion of T_4 to T_3	Inhibit iodination of tyrosine residues in thyroglobulin. Inhibit coupling of iodotyrosine residues to form T_3 and T_4	Inhibit iodination of tyrosine residues in thyroglobulin. Inhibit coupling of iodotyrosine residues to form T_3 and T_4	Inhibit organification. hormone release. Decreases size. vascularity of the hyperplastic gland	Destroy thyroid cells by emission of • particles
Dose	Dose 50-100mg TDS followed by 20-30mg BD-TDS for maintenance	Dose 5-15mg TDS followed by 2.5-10mg OD daily	Dose 5-10mg TDS followed by 5-15mg OD daily	lugol's iodine (5% solution in 10% Pot. Iodide solution) 5-10 drops/day	3-6 mcurie
Duration	Single dose acts for 4-8 hours	12-24 hours	12-24 hours		
Potency	Dose to dose less potent	About 3 times more potent	About 10 times more potent		
Transfer across placenta	Less	Large amounts	Large amounts		
Protein binding	Highly bound	Less bound	Less bound		
Metabolism	Metabolised in liver and excreted in urine. No active metabolite	Metabolised in liver and excreted in urine. Produces active metabolite methimazole	Metabolised in liver and excreted in urine. No active metabolite		
Use	Control thyrotoxicosis in Grave's disease, toxic nodular goitre	Control thyrotoxicosis in Grave's disease, toxic nodular goitre	Control thyrotoxicosis in Grave's disease, toxic nodular goitre	Preoperative preparation. Thyroid storm	Control hyperthyroidism in Grave's disease, toxic nodular goitre
Side effects	Granulocytopenia (rare), rashes, headache, nausea, jaundice, pain in the joints	Granulocytopenia (rare), rashes, headache, nausea, jaundice, pain in the joints	Granulocytopenia (rare), rashes, headache, nausea, jaundice, pain in the joints	Iodism, rash, swollen salivary glands, mucous membrane ulcerations, conjunctivitis, rhinorrhea, drug fever, metallic taste, bleeding disorders and, rarely, anaphylactoid reactions	Hypothyroidism

TABLE 4 Drugs used for hypothyroid patients

	l- thyroxine
Dose	50µg /day, may be increased to 100-200 µg/day
Indications	Hormone replacement therapy in cretinism, hypothyroidism, myxedema coma

Table 5 - Benzodiazepines

	Diazepam	Midazolam	Lorazepam
Mechanism of action	Facilitate action of GABA	Facilitate action of GABA	Facilitate action of GABA
Dose induction Maintenance Sedation	0.3-0.5 mg/kg 0.1 mg/kg 2 mg repeated	0.05-15 mg/kg 1µg/kg/min 0.07mg/kg i.m	0.1mg/kg 0.02 mg/kg 0.25 mg repeated
Onset	3-5 min	<3 min	10-20 min
Half life	20-66 hours	1-4 hours	10-20 hours
Metabolism	oxidation in liver to desmethyldiazepam, oxazepam	Hydroxylation in liver to 1-hydroxymidazolam, 4-hydroxymidazolam	Glucuronidation in liver
Actions	↓cerebral oxygen requirement, CBF, anticonvulasant, ↓ventilation, ↓BP,↑ Heart rate	↓cerebral oxygen requirement, CBF, anticonvulasant, ↓ventilation, ↓BP,↑ Heart rate	↓cerebral oxygen requirement, CBF, anticonvulasant, ↓ventilation, ↓BP,↑ Heart rate
Uses	Preoperative mediation, sedation, induction & maintenance of anaesthesia, anticonvulsant, treatment of local anaesthetic induced seizures, limits emergence from ketamine	Preoperative mediation, sedation, induction & maintenance of anaesthesia, limits emergence from ketamine	sedation, induction & maintenance of anaesthesia, anticonvulsant, limits emergence from ketamine
Side effects	Respiratory depression, thrombophlebitis drowsiness, fatigue	Respiratory depression	Respiratory depression, venous irritation, amnesia, drowsiness
Antagonist	Flumazenil	Flumazenil	Flumazenil

Table 6 - Anti epileptics

	Phenytoin	Carbamazepine	Sodium valproate
Group	Hydantoin	Iminostilbene	Aliphatic carboxylic acid

Mechanism of action	Stabilizes influence on neuronal membrane by ↑ inactive state of sodium channels	Modifies maximum electroshock seizures by ↑ inactive state of sodium channels, ↑ADH action on renal tubules	↑ inactive state of sodium channels, ↑ calcium mediated T current, ↓degradation of GABA
Dose	300 mg/d,	15–25 mg/kg/d	200 mg tds
Half life	24 hours	36 hours	10-15 hours
Metabolism	In liver	In liver	In liver
Uses	partial seizures, generalized tonic-clonic seizures, trigeminal neuralgia	partial seizures, generalized tonic-clonic seizures, trigeminal neuralgia, some patients of mania	Absence seizures, generalized tonic-clonic seizures, myoclonic & atonic seizures, manic – depressive psychosis
Adverse effects	Nystagmus, loss of smooth extraocular pursuit movements, Diplopia, ataxia, Gingival hyperplasia, hirsutism, megaloblastic anemia	mild gastrointestinal upsets, unsteadiness, Diplopia, ataxia, aplastic anemia, agranulocytosis, skin rash	mild gastrointestinal upsets, ataxia, tremor, alopecia, rash, thrombocytopenia, fulminant hepatitis

Table 7 -Drugs used in mental illness

	Chlorpromazine	Lithium	Clozapine	Amitriptyline	Fluoxetine
Group	Anti psychotic, Others – trifluperazine, haloperidol, pimozide	Mood stabilising agent	Anti psychotic	Tricyclic antidepressant	Selective serotonin reuptake inhibitor
Mechanism of action	Blocks D_2 receptor	Replaces Na+ affecting ionic fluxes, ↓release of noradrenaline & dopamine, ↓ADH action	$5HT_2, D_4$, α_1 blocking action	Inhibit uptake of NA & 5 HT	Inhibit uptake of 5 HT
Dose	100-800mg/day	0.5 mEq/kg/d conc.0.5-1.2 mEq/l	25-300mg/day	50-200mg/d	20-60mg/d

Half life	30 hours	20 hours		31–46 hours	24–96 hours
Actions	Neuroleptic syndrome, ↓irrational behaviour, ↓anxiety & agitation, anticholinergic action, ↓BP,↑HR, ↑prolactin release	↑sleep time in mania, suppresses manic episodes	Suppresses positive & negative symptoms of schizophrenia, same as Chlorpromazine	Sedation, antimuscuranic action, elevate mood, ↑HR, postural hypotension, arrhythmias,	No sedation or antimuscuranic action
Metabolism	In liver	Unchanged in urine	In liver	In liver to Nortriptyline	In liver to Norfluoxetine
Indications	Psychoses, mania, anxiety, alcoholic hallucinations	Acute manic episode, prophylaxis of MDI, recurrent neuropsychiatric illness	Psychoses, mania, anxiety, alcoholic hallucinations	Depression, prophylaxis of migraine, neuropathic pain	Prophylaxis of recurrent depression, obsessicve compulsive disorders
Side effects	Drowsiness, seizures in epileptics, hypotension, dry mouth, extrapyramidal disturbance, hypersensitivity reactions	Nausea, vomiting, thrist, polyuria, tremors, motor incoordination, arrhythmia, diabetes inspidius, goitre	Agranulocytosis, sedation, hypersalivation, unstable BP, tachycardia, myocarditis	Dry mouth, sedation, ↑ appetite, seizures, arrhythmias, postural hypotension	Anxiety, insomnia, dyskinesia, nausea, headache, hypernatremia,

other tricyclic antidepressants used- imipramine, trimipramine, clemipramine, doxepin, dothepin
MAO inhibitors – phenelzine, isocarboxid, tranylcypromine, maclobemide

Table 8 - Drugs used in gastrointestinal system

Drugs	Ondansetron	Metoclopramide	Ranitidine	Pantoprazole	Granisetron
Group	5 HT_3 antagonist	Prokinetic	H_2 antagonist	Proton pump inhibitor	5 HT_3 antagonist
Mechanism of action	Inhibit the ion channel of 5 HT_3 receptor	Dopamine antagonism, cholinomimetic, 5 HT_3 antagonist	Competitive antagonist at H_2 receptors	Inactivates the enzyme H^+K^+ ATPase to decrease secretion	Inhibit the ion channel of 5 HT_3 receptor
Dose	0.06 mg/kg IV	10 mg IM, oral tds	150 mg bd oral, 50mgIV 6-8 hrly	40 mg od	0.04mg/kg IV
Metabolism	In liver	In liver	In liver	In liver	in liver
Actions	Antiemetic- inhibits Chemoreceptor Trigger Zone	Promotes gastroduodenal peristalsis, speeds gastric emptying, antiemetic	Block stimuli induced gastric secretion & histamine induced cardiac stimulation & bronchial relaxation	Inhibits secretion gastric acid	Antiemetic- inhibits Chemoreceptor Trigger Zone
Indications	Chemotherapy induced & post operative vomiting	Vomiting gastroesophageal reflux disease, dyspepsia	Peptic ulcers, stress ulcers, ZE syndrome, GERD	Peptic ulcers, ZE syndrome, GERD	Chemotherapy induced & post operative vomiting
Side effects	Headache, mild constipation	Sedation, diarrhoea, muscle dystonia, parkinsonism, galactorrhoea	Headache, diarrhoea, dizziness, rash, hepatic injury	Diarrhoea, nausea, headache, abdominal pain, leucopenia, hepatic dysfunction, atrophic gastritis	Headache, mild constipation

Table 9 - Drugs used in obstetrics

Oxytocin – hormone produced by posterior pituitary, also prepared synthetically.
    Stimulates uterine contractions in pregnant patients
        To induce labour- solution of 10mU/ml is used @1-2mU/min.
        To treat uterine atony – upto 40mU/min used
    Side effects- decrease in blood pressure, flushing, water intoxication
Ergometrine – ergot alkaloid, stimulates uterine contractions,
        Dose – for uterine contraction 0.2 – 1 mg i.m or 0.1-0.5 mg i.v
        For migraine – 0.5 mg orally
    Side effects – hypertension, acute pulmonary oedema, cerebral oedema, convulsion

Phosphodiasterase III inhibitors

Mechanism of action- inhibit degradation of cAMP increasing calcium entry leading to positive inotropic action & systemic, pulmonary vasodilatory effects
Use: Right ventricular & biventricular failure. Improves myocardial diastolic relaxation enhancing left ventricular filling & coronary perfusion. Dose: milrinone–50mg/kg followed by 0.5mg/kg/min i.v amrinone – 0.75 to 1.5 mg/kg followed by 10mg/kg/min I.v

Table 10-Vitamin K
fat soluble vitamin required for synthesis of clotting factors – prothrombin, VII, IX, X

Requirement – 50-100mg/day

deficiency- occurs due to obstructive jaundice, liver disease, malabsoption leads to bleeding tendency.

Use – prophylaxis & treatment of bleeding due to deficiency of clotting factors.

Toxicity – flushing, breathlessness, fall in BP, kernicterus in newborn

Table 11-Anticoagulants

	Heparin	Oral anticoagulants
Mechanism of action	Binds to antithrombin & inactivates factor X, XII, XI, IX	Inhibits vitamin K epoxide reductase & vitamin K reductase
Monitor	APTT- 1.5-2.5 times predrug value, ACT	INR - 2.0-3.0
Dose	Prophylaxis against venous thromboembolism - 5000 IU s.c every 8 to 12 hours Treatment of venous thromboembolism - 5000 IU followed by 30000U every 24 hours infusion Treatment of MI - 5000 IU followed by 24000U every 24 hours infusion Low molecular weight heparin- enoxaparin exhibits less binding to endothelial cells leading to less bleeding tendency	Warfarin - 15 mg first day followed by 20 mg on second day then 2.5 to 10 mg Dicoumarol - 200 mg on first two days then 25-200 mg/day Phenindione 300 mg followed by 200 mg on next day then 25-200 mg/day
Side effects	Haemorrhage, thrombocytopenia, allergic reactions, hypotension, altered protein binding Antagonist - protamine 1mg for every 100 U of heparin	

Table 12: Drug Interactions

	Drugs affecting action	Effect
Cardiac glycosides- digitalis	Suxamethonium chloride, sympathomimetic amines	Ventricular arrhythmias
	Halothane, neostigmine	Excessive bradycardia
	Calcium	Potentiates arrythmogenic effect
	Broad spectrum antibiotics	Enhance toxicity
Quinidine	Muscle relaxants	Prolongs the duration of block
Antihypertensives - ACE inhibitors	Sodium nitroprusside	Reduce tachyphylaxis
Glyceryl trinitrate	Antimuscarine agents	Reduce absorption of sublingual nitrates
Clonidine	Opioids	Decrease requirements
	Local anaesthetics	Potentiates effect
Ganglionic blocking drugs	Neuromuscular blockers	Prolong and intensify effect
Calcium channel blockers	Carbamazepine	Serum level rises
	Bupivacaine	Cardiotoxicity increases
	Volatile anaesthetics	Additive effect on conduction
	Neuromuscular blockers	Increase potency
β blockers	Halothane	Sudden cardiovascular collapse may occur
	Warfarin, digoxin, quinidine	Reduced clearance
Diuretics- thiazides	Digitalis	Increase toxicity
	Neuromuscular blockers	Potentiates effect
	lithium	Impaired renal clearance
Spironolactone	Suxamethonium chloride	Arrhythmias
Phenothiazines	Barbiturates	Cross tolerance
Analgesics - narcotics	Depolarising relaxants	Susceptible
	Non depolarising relaxants	resistant
Anticonvulsant - phenytoin	benzodiazepines	Increased levels of phenytoin
	Folic acid	Decreased levels of phenytoin
	Non depolarising relaxants	Resistance to actions
Antidepressants-tricyclic antidepressants	MAO inhibitors	Hypertensive crisis
	Halothane	Ventricular arrhythmias
MAO inhibitors	Sympathomimetic drugs	Exaggerated response
	Sedatives, hypnotics, narcotic analgesics.	Cardiovascular depression, respiratory depression, convulsion, pyrexia
Antipsychotics	Sedatives	Potentiated
Lithium	Relaxants	Effect potentiated
Anticoagulants	Barbiturates	Anticoagulant effect reduced
	Salicylates, antimicrobials	Effect potentiated
Volatile anaesthetic agents- halothane	Adrenaline	Arrhythmias
	Phenobarbitone	Halothane induced hepatitis
	Non depolarising relaxants	Effect potentiated
Induction agents-thiopentone	Contrast media, sulphonamides	free drug
	Ethanol, opioids, antihistamines, CNS depressants	Potentiate sedative effects
Ketamine	Non depolarising muscle relaxants	Potentiated
	Theophylline	Seizures
	Diazepam	Attenuates ketamine's sympathetic effects
	Lithium	Duration prolonged
Etomidate	Fentanyl	Prolongs elimination half life
	Opioids	Decrease myoclonus
Propofol	Opioids	Increased concentrations of opioids

References
1. Miller J. Anesthesia 6th Ed. Philadelphia, Churchill-Livingstone, 2004.
2. Kumar P. Textbook of Anaesthesia. Hyderabad, Paras Pub Med ,2007
3. Pramod Kumar.Textbook of anaesthesia and analgesia. Part 1: Basic sciences. Ist Edn, Amazon Kindle, New York,2018

Chapter 15 Generic Medicine

A generic drug is a **pharmaceutical drug** that is equivalent to a brand-name product in dosage, strength, route of administration, quality, performance, and intended use. This means any drug marketed under its chemical name without advertising or to the chemical makeup of a drug rather than the brand name under which the drug is sold.

This initiative by Govt of India to promote generic medicine will provide quality drugs at very low prices, removing a great burden on patients of this region. Medical council of India also has made it compulsory for all doctors to write only generic drugs to each and end every patient. Given below is an introduction to generic drugs which is an initiative of Government of India

Although they may not be associated with a particular company, generic drugs are usually subject to government regulations in the countries where they are dispensed. They are labeled with the name of the manufacturer and a generic **international nonproprietary name** of the drug. A generic drug must contain the same **active ingredients** as the original brand-name formulation. The U.S. Food and Drug Administration (FDA) requires that generics be identical to, or within an acceptable **bioequivalent** range of, their brand-name counterparts with respect to **pharmacokinetic** and **pharmacodynamic** properties.

In most cases, generic products become available after the **patent protections** afforded to a drug's original developer expire. Once generic drugs enter the market, competition often leads to substantially lower prices for both the original brand-name product and its generic equivalents. In most countries, patents give 20 years of protection. However, many countries and regions, such as the European Union and the United States, may grant up to five years of additional protection ("restoration") if manufacturers meet specific goals, such as conducting **clinical trials** for paediatric patients. Manufacturers, wholesalers, insurers, and drug stores can each increase prices at various stages of production and distribution.[1]

In 2014, according to an analysis by the Generic Pharmaceutical Association, generic drugs accounted for 88% of the 4.3 billion prescriptions filled in the United States.[2]

Economics

Generic drugs are usually sold for significantly lower prices than their branded equivalents and at lower **profit margins**. One reason for this is that competition increases among producers when a drug is no longer protected by patents. Generic companies incur fewer costs in creating generic drugs—only the cost of manufacturing, without the costs of **drug discovery** and **drug development**—and are therefore able to maintain **profitability** at a lower price. The prices are often low enough for users in less-prosperous countries to afford them. For example, Thailand has imported millions of doses of a generic version of the blood-thinning drug **Plavix** (used to help prevent heart attacks) from India, the leading manufacturer of generic drugs, at a cost of 3 US cents per dose. Generic drug companies may also receive the benefit of the previous marketing efforts of the brand-name company, including advertising, presentations by drug representatives, and distribution of free samples. Many drugs introduced by generic manufacturers have already been on the market for a decade or more and may already be well known to patients and providers, although often under their branded name.

Regulation

Most nations require generic drug manufacturers to prove that their formulations are bioequivalent to their brand-name counterparts. Bioequivalence does not mean generic drugs must be exactly the same as the brand-name product (pharmaceutical equivalent). Chemical differences may exist; a different salt or ester may be used. However, the therapeutic effect of the drug must be the same. Most small molecule drugs are accepted as bioequivalent if their pharmacokinetic parameters of area under the curve (AUC) and maximum concentration (C_{max}) are within a 90% confidence interval of 80–125%; most approved generics are well within this limit. For more complex products—such as inhalers, patch delivery systems, liposomal preparations, or bio similar drugs—demonstrating pharmaco dynamic or clinical equivalence is more challenging.

United States

Before a company can market a generic drug, it needs to file an Abbreviated New Drug Application (ANDA) with the Food and Drug Administration, seeking to demonstrate therapeutic equivalence to a previously approved "reference-listed drug" and proving that it can manufacture the drug safely and consistently. For an ANDA to be approved, the FDA requires the bioequivalence of a generic drug to be between 80% and 125% of the innovator product. This range is part of a statistical calculation, and does not mean that generic drugs are allowed to differ from their brand-name counterparts by up to 25 percent.[1]

The FDA evaluated 2,070 studies conducted between 1996 and 2007 that compared the absorption of brand-name and generic drugs into a person's body. The average difference in absorption between the generic and the brand-name drug was 3.5 percent, comparable to the difference between two batches of a brand-name drug. Generic versions of biologic drugs, or biosimilars, require clinical trials for immunogenicity in addition to tests establishing bioequivalency. These products cannot be entirely identical because of batch-to-batch variability and their biological nature, and they are subject to extra rules.

China

Generic drug production is a large part of the pharmaceutical industry in China. Western observers have said that China lacks administrative protection for patents. However, entry to the World Trade Organization has brought a stronger patent system.

Acceptance

A series of scandals around the approval of generic drugs in the late 1980s shook public confidence in generic drugs; there were several instances in which companies obtained bioequivalence data fraudulently, by using the branded drug in their tests instead of their own product, and a congressional investigation found corruption at the FDA, where employees were accepting bribes to approve some generic companies' applications and delaying or denying others. Some generic drugs are viewed with suspicion by doctors. For example, warfarin (Coumadin) has a narrow therapeutic window and requires frequent blood tests to make sure patients do not have a sub therapeutic or a toxic level. A study performed in Ontario showed that replacing Coumadin with generic warfarin was safe, but many physicians are not comfortable with their patients taking branded generic equivalents. In some countries (for example, Australia) where a drug is prescribed under more than one brand name, doctors may choose not to allow pharmacists to substitute a brand different from the one prescribed unless the consumer requests it.

Recalls

In 2007, North Carolina Public Radio's The People's Pharmacy began reporting on consumers complaints that generic versions of bupropion (Wellbutrin) were yielding unexpected effects. Subsequently, Impax Laboratories's 300 mg extended-release tablets, marketed by Teva Pharmaceutical Industries, were withdrawn from the US market after the FDA determined in 2012 that they were not bioequivalent.

Litigation

Two women, each claiming to have suffered severe medical complications from a generic version of **metoclopramide**, lost their Supreme Court appeal on June 23, 2011. In a 5-4 ruling in **PLIVA, Inc. V. Mensing**, in which the court held that generic companies cannot be held liable for information, or the lack of information, on the originator's label.[1]

India

The **Indian government** began encouraging more drug manufacturing by Indian companies in the early 1960s, and with the Patents Act in 1970. The Patents Act removed composition patents for foods and drugs, and though it kept process patents, these were shortened to a period of five to seven years. The resulting lack of patent protection created a niche in both the Indian and global markets that Indian companies filled by reverse-engineering new processes for manufacturing low-cost drugs. The code of ethics issued by the **Medical Council of India** in 2002 calls for physicians to prescribe drugs by their generic names only.

One Key requirement for generic makers is to submit bio-equivalent (BE) studies. A BE study is a process where companies have to test their generic products as against the innovator's product for their effectiveness. In India, the requirement of BE study is a grey area.

S. Srinivas of the All India Drugs Action Network, an organization working to improve access to drugs, warned about doctors, fear mongering that non-branded medicines are of poor quality. He said "The argument that all generic are of poor quality and all branded drugs are great is misleading. For this proposal to work, the government not only needs to ban the use of brands completely, but also make sure chemists have full stock of generic medicines."

One the other hand, public health activists say this is how India should move forward as far as medicines are concerned. "The will be path-breaking move if it comes through. The government needs to ensure chemists do not stock highly expensive medicines and state drug regulator should ensure quality," said Leena Menghaney of Doctors without Borders, an aid organization.

Prime Minister Narendra stated that doctors visit illegible prescription which leads to pharmacist selling a drug of brand where he gets maximum profit margin. There are stories of a nexus between pharmacist and doctors where higher percentage of commission (upto 30-40% in case of stents, superspeciality products) increase the cost of treatment many folds. There has been a strong opposition from drug manufacture and physician lobby against generic drug prescription. Government has taken care of quality test of these generic drugs under Pradhan Mantri Jan Aushidhi Priyojna where the quality control of each drug is being under taken.[3]

Inspite of all arguments against generic drugs, the fact remains that each citizen has right to a quality drug which is affordable. He also has a right to choose a particular drug brand.

References

1. Generic Drugs, Centre, U.S. Food and Drug Administration. January 12, 2010. Retrieved 2010-02-03.
2. Doctors to prescribe generic drugs only or face action, says MCI BY PTI | APR 22, 2017.
3. PM Narendra Modi's proposal over generic drugs isn't a new one BY DIVYA RAJAGOPAL, ET BUREAU APR 21, 2017.

Chapter 16   ASA Guidelines on labeling of pharmaceuticals for use in anesthesiology

STATEMENT ON CREATING LABELS OF PHARMACEUTICALS FOR USE IN ANESTHESIOLOGY

Committee of Origin: Equipment and Facilities

(Approved by the ASA House of Delegates on October 27, 2004, and last amended on October 28, 2015)

Rationale:

The practice of anesthesiology requires administering a wide variety of potent medications. These medications are often given in high acuity situations and in environments with poor visibility and multiple distractions. Medications with widely differing actions, such as muscle relaxants, vasopressors, and vasodilators, are often used in the course of a single anesthetic, at times simultaneously. It has been recognized for some time that perioperative medication errors are a significant source of morbidity and, rarely, mortality.[1-4] Interest in medication errors has extended to regulatory agencies, the federal government, and the general public.

Medications are often selected based upon the location and visual features of the container/syringe. The recognition and identification of an object depends on shape, color, brightness, and contrast. As these elements become increasingly distinctive, identification of the object becomes faster and more accurate.[5-7] Identification of the medication is verified by reading the label. Therefore, although multiple factors contribute to medication errors, consistency and clarity of pharmaceutical and syringe labeling, in accordance with human factors, are important elements in their prevention. ASTM has come out with their own standards regarding how best to label pharmaceutical containing syringes and vials.[8-9] There are some minor differences in the standard colors as designated by ASTM and ISO. This Statement will provide the standards of each and highlight where differences exist.

Statement:

The primary consideration in the design of labels for syringes and drug infusion bags should be patient safety and the reduction of medication errors. This is particularly true for the potent medications used in the practice of anesthesiology. Therefore, the ASA supports the manufacture and use of labels meeting the following standards, which are consistent with those established by ASTM International (ASTM), the International Organization for Standardization (ISO), and the Institute for Safe Medication Practices (ISMP):

1. **Label Content**: The drug's generic name and concentration for syringe labels, and the total volume or contents for an infusion bag should be the most prominent items displayed on the label of each syringe or infusion bag containing pharmaceuticals for use in the practice of anesthesiology.

2. **Font**: The text on the label should be designed to enhance the legibility, of the drug name and concentration as recommended in ASTM D4267, Standard Specification for Labels for Small-Volume (100 ml or less) Parenteral Drug Containers and D6398, Standard Practice to Enhance Identification of Drug

Names on Labels, and ISO 26825:2008, Anaesthetic and respiratory equipment – User-applied labels for syringes containing drugs used during anaesthesia – Colour, design and performance. These standards include recommendations for font size, extra space for separation around the drug name, and use of additional emphasis for the initial syllable, or a distinctive syllable, of similar drug names.

3. **Contrasting Background**: Maximum contrast between the text and background should be provided by high-contrast color combinations as specified in Section 6.3.1 of ASTM

D6398-08. This minimizes the impact of color blindness:

Text	Background
Black	White
Blue	Yellow
White	Blue
Blue	White

4. **Color:** Nine classes of drugs commonly used in the practice of anesthesiology have a standard background color established for user-applied syringe labels by ASTM D4774-11, Standard Specifications for User Applied Drug Labels in Anesthesiology and ISO 26825:2008 (only eight, copper has not been added).

	PMS [a]	ASTM [b] - RGB		ISO [c] - RGB
Induction Agents	Process Yellow C	255.255.0		255.255.0
Benzodiazepines and Tranquilizers	Orange 151	255.102.0		255.102.0
Benzodiazepine Antagonists	Orange 151 / White Diagonal Stripes	255.102.0		255.102.0
Muscle Relaxants	Florescent Red 805 [d]	255.114.118		
	Florescent Red 811 [e]			253.121.86
	Warm Red [f]			245.64.41
Muscle Relaxant Antagonists	Florescent Red / White Diagonal Stripes	255.114.118		253.121.86
Opioid/Narcotics	Blue 297	133.199.227		133.199.227
Opioid/Narcotic Antagonists	Blue 297 / White Diagonal Stripes	133.199.227		133.199.227
Major Tranquilizers and Anti-Emetics	Salmon 156	237.194.130		237.194.130
Vasopressors	Violet 256	222.191.217		222.191.217
Hypotensive Agents	Violet 256/White Diagonal Stripes	222.191.217		222.191.217
Local Anesthetics	Gray 401	194.184.171		194.184.171
Anticholinergic Agents	Green 367	163.217.99		163.217.99
Beta Blockers	Copper 876U	176.135.112		NA [g]
	White	255.255.255		255.255.255

a - Pantone Matching System
b - ASTM International; prior to 2001 it was the American Society for Testing and Materials
c - International Organization for Standardization
d - Designated by ASTM International
e - Designated by ISO
f - Designated by ISO as an alternative if Florescent Red cannot be printed
g - ISO has not designated a color for Beta Blockers

IMPORTANT — The colors represented in this electronic file are not intended to be used for color matching.

RGB (Red, Green, Blue) is used only for digital (computer based) designs. Any design created with an RGB color profile must be converted to CMYK (Cyan, Magenta, Yellow, blacK) or PMS color codes before printing. As a rule of thumb, you should only use RGB when designing for computer-based applications.

5. **Label Enhancements to Reduce Drug Administration Errors:**

- **Bar coding**: Essential information, including the drug's generic name and concentration could be bar coded at a location on the label which will not interfere with the label's legibility, as specified in Section 8 of ASTM D6398.

- **Label material** shall allow the user to write information on it using a ball-point pen or felt-tip marker without smudging or blurring as specified in Section 2.3 of ISO 26825:2008.

- **Printing:** All printing is in black bold type with the exception of succinylcholine and epinephrine which are printed against the background color as reverse plate letters within a black bar running from edge to edge of the label.

Tall Man Letters

The FDA Office of Generic Drugs requested manufacturers of sixteen look-alike name pairs to voluntarily revise the appearance of their established names in order to minimize medication errors resulting from look-alike confusion. Letters from the FDA encouraged manufacturers to revise labels and labeling that visually differentiated their established names with the use of "Tall Man" letters. The following are Tall Man drug names from lists of easily confused medications compiled by the FDA and the ISMP that may be administered by the anesthesia care team during a procedure.

ChlorproMAZINE	DiphenhydrAMINE	DOBUTamine	DOPamine
ePHEDrine	EPINEPHrine	fentaNYL	HydrALAZINE
HYDROmorphone	HydrOXYzine	NiCARdipine	SUFentanil

Useful Websites (last accessed May 2015):

For referenced ASTM International standards, visit the ASTM Website Reading Room at: http://www.astm.org/READINGLIBRARY/
or, send an email to ASTM customer service at: service@astm.org
For referenced ISO standards, visit the ISO (International Organization for Standardization) Website at: http://www.iso.org/iso/home.html
FDA Name Differentiation Project
http://www.fda.gov/Drugs/DrugSafety/MedicationErrors/ucm164587.htm
FDA/ISMP Tall Man Letters
https://www.ismp.org/tools/tallmanletters.pdf
Institute for Safe Medication Practices (ISMP) Syringe Label Guidelines
http://www.ismp.org/tools/guidelines/labelFormats/Injectable.asp
Error-prone abbreviations
http://www.ismp.org/Tools/errorproneabbreviations.pd

Chapter 17. ASA Guidelines security of medications in the operating room

STATEMENT ON SECURITY OF MEDICATIONS IN THE OPERATING ROOM

(Approved by the ASA Executive Committee in October 2003, and last amended by the ASA House of Delegates on October 16, 2013)

Preamble

A secure environment of care is needed for medication safety. Medication safety includes the security of oral, sublingual, parenteral, and inhaled drugs used for elective and emergency patient care. A secure area ensures the integrity of anesthesia machines as well as other equipment and materials. Security of medications in the operating room suite is essential for patient safety.

Recommended Policies

1. Access to operating room suites must be strictly limited to authorized persons.
2. All Schedule 3 and 4 narcotic medications must be kept in locked enclosed areas when not under the direct control of an anesthesia professional.
3. Anesthesia professionals must have immediate access to drugs required for emergency patient care. Procedures designed to prevent unauthorized access to such drugs must be consistent with this imperative for patient safety.
4. Anesthesia carts and anesthesia machines may remain unlocked, and non-controlled* medications may be left in or on top of unlocked anesthesia carts or anesthesia machines immediately prior to, during, and immediately following surgical cases in an operating room, so long as there are authorized operating room personnel in the OR suite.

Rationale

A. Because the operating room suite is a limited-access secure location, it is safe practice for anesthesia professionals to leave non-controlled* medications on the top of their anesthesia carts or anesthesia machines for brief periods (e.g., while going to a nearby holding area to bring a patient into the operating room).
B. At the end of anesthesia cases, when patients are particularly vulnerable, anesthesia professionals dedicate full attention to their patients. This vulnerable period extends from the time the patient emerges from anesthesia until the anesthesia professional transports the patient to a recovery area (e.g., post anesthesia care unit, intensive care unit, etc.). If drugs are locked up during this vulnerable period, provider access to drugs required for emergency patient care is obstructed. Furthermore, requiring anesthesia professionals to divert attention from patients in order to lock non-controlled* medications in anesthesia carts during the period between emergence from anesthesia and transport of patients out of the operating room jeopardizes patient safety. Therefore, locking non-controlled* medications at this point in the anesthetic should not be required.
C. It is necessary and safe practice for non-controlled* medications to be set up for emergency cases (e.g., in obstetrics and trauma) and made secure in a drawer or cupboard "locked" by a tamper-evident device that can easily be broken by authorized

persons. Locks requiring knowledge of a combination or possession of a physical key jeopardize patient safety.

D. It is necessary and safe practice for emergency anesthesia drugs (e.g., dantrolene for the treatment of malignant hyperthermia) to be kept in a dedicated emergency cart or cupboard and made secure ("locked") by a tamper-evident device that can easily be broken by authorized persons. Locks requiring knowledge of a combination or possession of a physical key jeopardize patient safety.

*The term "non-controlled" refers to medications that are not Schedule II-V narcotics.

Annexure 1 ALGORITHMS FOR MECHANISM OF ACTION OF DRUGS

Annexture 1 Mechanism of action of drugs

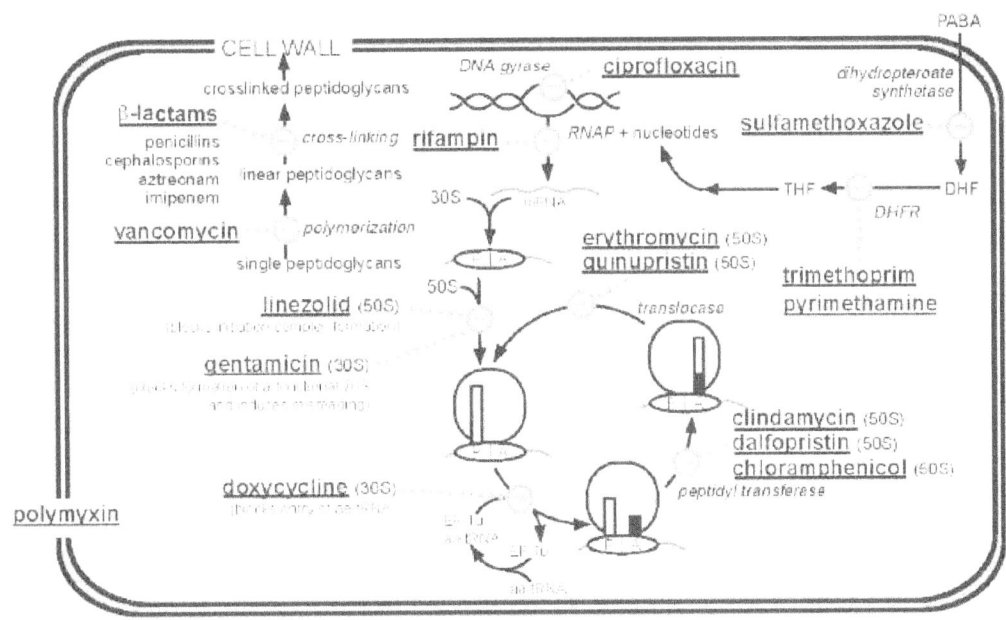

Site of Action of Insulin, Pramlintide

INSULIN / Pramlintide

Preparation type	Use	Examples
Rapidly acting	Prandial bolus to cover extra requirements after food	Aspart, glulisine, lispro, regular, crystalline zinc insulin (CZI)
Intermediate or long acting	Basal supplementation to suppress glucose production and maintain normoglycemia in the fasting state	NPH (neutral protamine Hagedorn), lente, ultralente, detemir, glargine

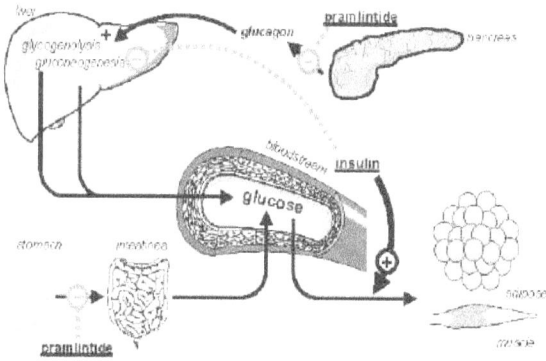

Site of Action of Oral Anti Diabetic Drugs

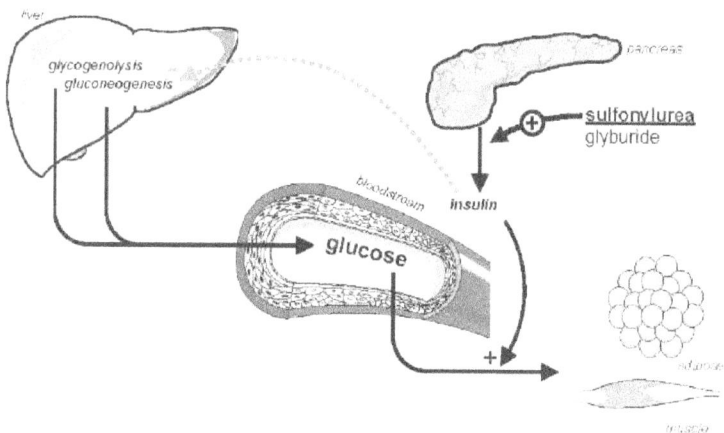

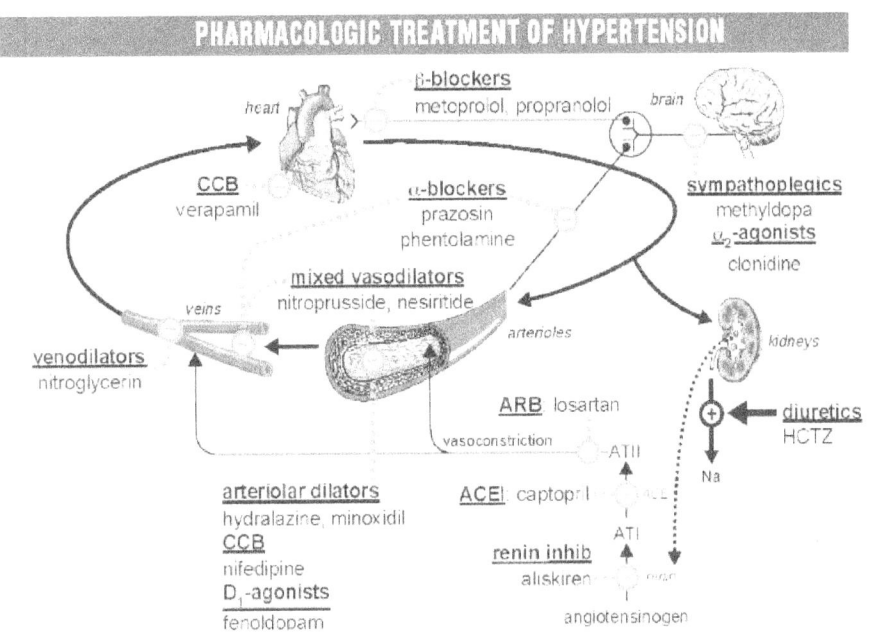

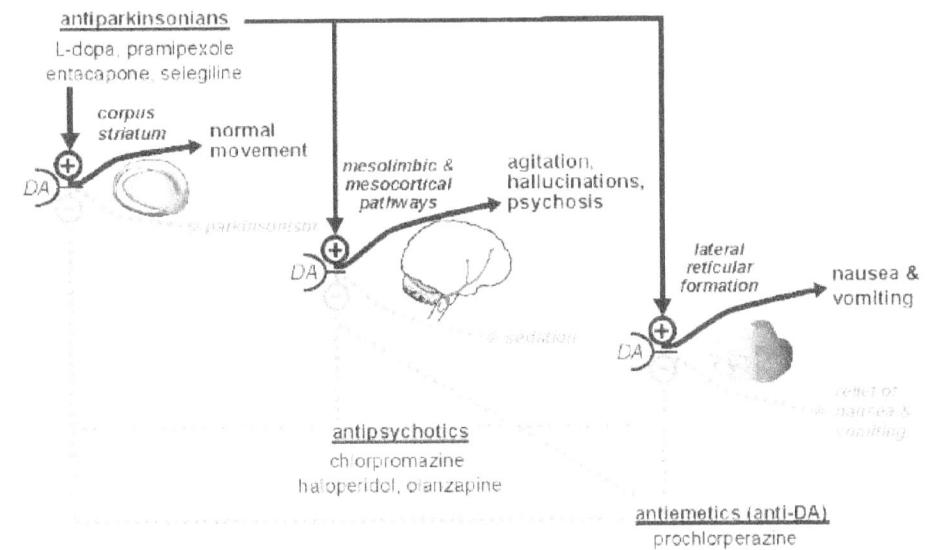

ANTIEPILEPTIC AGENTS

Inhibitory neuronal projection
- Vigabatrin
- Tiagabine
- Benzodiazepines
- Barbiturates
- Topiramate

Excitatory neuronal projection
- Phenytoin
- Carbamazepine
- Valproic Acid
- Lamotrigine
- Felbamate
- Topiramate
- Zonisamide
- Topiramate
- Felbamate

Tubular Filtration of Electrolytes & Spironolectone

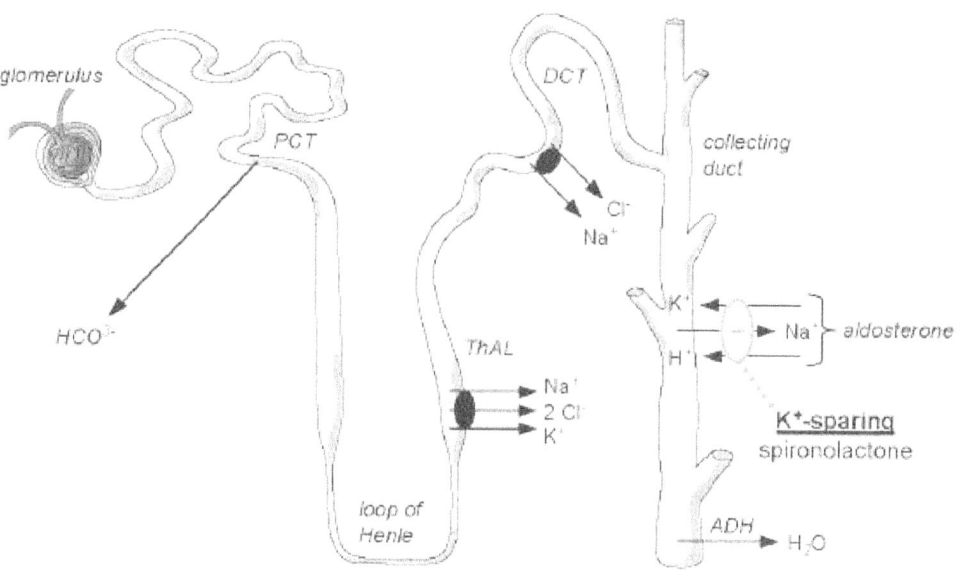

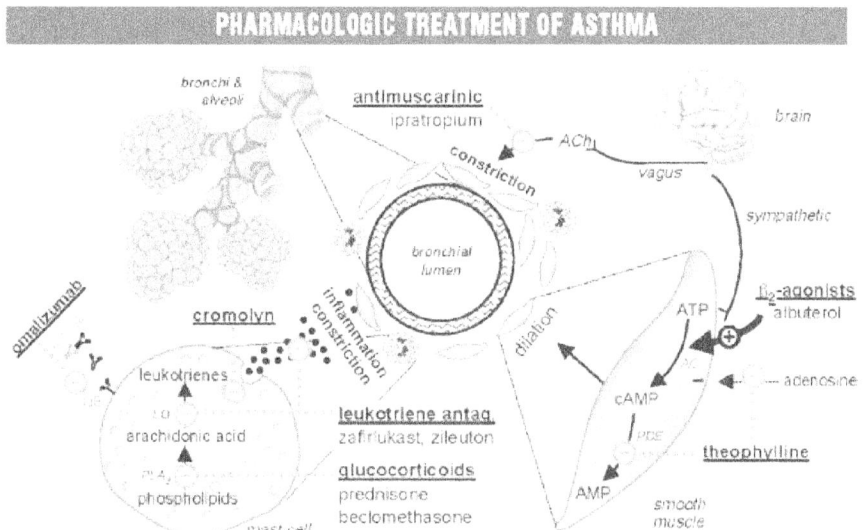

Annexture 2   Pharmacology Mnemonics

Pharmacology Mnemonics
1. Sulfonamides: common characteristics SULFA:
   S-Steven-Johnson syndrome/ Skin rash / Solubility low
   U-Urine precipitation/ Useful for UTIL-Large spectrum (gram positives and negatives)
   F-Folic acids synthesis blocker (as well as synthesis of nucleic acids)
   A-Analog of PABA
2. Diuretics: groups "L OTCAN":
   L-Loop diuretics
   O-Osmotics
   T-Thiazides
   C-Carbonic anhydrase inhibitors
   A-Aldosterone inhibitors
   N-Na (sodium) channel blockers
3. Tuberculosis treatment- PRIEST":
   P-Pyrazinamide
   R-Rifampin
   I-Isoniazid (INH)
   E-Ethambutol
   St-Streptomycin
4. Aminoglycosides: common characteristics- AMINO:
   Active Against Aerobic gram negative
   Mechanism of resistance are Modifying enzymes
   Inhibit protein synthesis by binding to 30S subunit
   Nephrotoxic
   Ototoxic
5. Cocaine: cardiovascular effect COcaine causes blood vessels to Constrict.
6. Thalidomide: effect on cancer cells "Thalidomide
   makes the blood vessels hide":
   Use thalidomide to stop cancer cells from growing new blood vessels.
7. Carbamazepine (CBZ): use CBZ:
   C-Cranial Nerve V (trigeminal) neuralgia
   B-Bipolar disorder
   Z-Zeisures
8. Warfarin: interactions ACADEMIC QACS:
   A-Amiodarone
   C-Cimetidine
   A-Aspirin
   D-Dapsone
   E-Erythromycin
   M-Metronidazole
   I-Indomethacin
   C-Clofibrates
   Q-Quinidine
   A-Azapropazone
   C-Ciprofloxacin
   S-Statins

9. Morphine: side-effects MORPHINE:
   M-Myosis
   O-Out of it (sedation)
   R-Respiratory depression
   P-Pneumonia (aspiration)
   H-Hypotension
   I-Infrequency (constipation, urinary retention)
   N-Nausea
   E-Emesis
10. Tricyclicantidepressants sideffects- TCA'S:
    T-Thrombocytopenia
    C-Cardiac (arrhythmia, MI, stroke)
    A-Anticholinergic (tachycardia, urinary retention)
    S-Seizures
11. Corticosteroids: adverse side effects- CUSHINGS BAD MD:
    C-Cataracts
    U-Up all night (sleep disturbances)
    S-Suppression of HPA axis
    H-Hypertension/ buffalo Hump
    I-Infections
    N-Necrosis (avascular)
    G-Gain weight
    S-Striae
    B-Bone loss (osteoporosis)
    A-Acne
    D-Diabetes
    M-Myopathy, moon faces
    D-Depression and emotional changes
12. Microtubules: drugs that act on microtubules.TMT GVC:
    T-Thiabendazole
    M-Mebendazole
    T-Taxol
    G-Griseofulvin
    V-Vincristine/ Vinblastine
    C-Colchicine
    BromoCRYPTine is a DOPamine agonist.
13. Beta blockers: members "The NEPAL PM
    T-Timolol
    N-Nadolol
    E-Esmolol
    P-Pindolol
    A-Atenolol
    L-Labetalol
    P-Propranolol
    M-Metoprolol
14. Insulin: mixing regular insulin and NPH-ANR DRN.
    Air into NPH
    Air into Regular

Draw up Regular
Draw up NPH
15. Parasympathetic vs. sympathetic neurotransmitters "No sympathy for a Pair of Aces":
Norepinephren is secreted in by the Sympathetic nervous system while Acetylcholine is secreted in the Parasympathetic nervous system.
16. Benzodiazepines: extrahepatic metabolism-LOT
L-Lorazepam
17. O-Oxazepam
T-Temazepam
18. Guanethidine: mechanism GuaNEthidine prevents NE (norepinephrine) release.
19. Opiods: mu receptor effects- MD CARES:
M-Miosis
D-Dependency
C-Constipation
A-Analgesics
R-Respiratory depression
E-Euphoria
S-Sedation
20. Adrenoceptors: vasomotor function of alpha vs. Beta- ABCD:
Alpha = Constrict.
Beta = Dilate.
21. Beta 1 selective blockers-MEA
22. M-Metropolol
23. E-Esmolol
A-Atenolol
24. Atropine use: tachycardia or bradycardia "A goes with B":
Atropine used clinically to treat Bradycardia.
25. Cancer drugs: time of action between DNA->mRNA- ABCDEF:
A-Alkylating agents
B-Bleomycin
C-Cisplastin
D-Dactinomycin/ Doxorubicin
E-Etoposide
F-Flutamide and other steroids or their antagonists (eg tamoxifen,leuprolide)
26. Busulfan: features ABCDEF:
A-Alkylating agent
B-Bone marrow suppression s/e
C-CML indication
D-Dark skin (hyperpigmentation) s/e
E-Endrocrine insufficiency (adrenal) s/e
F-Fibrosis (pulmonary) s/e
27. Tricyclic antidepressants- CIA
28. C-Clomipramine
I-Imipramine
A-Amitrptyline

29. Torsades de Pointes: drugs causing- APACHE:
    A-Amiodarone
    P-Procainamide
    A-Arsenium
    C-Cisapride
    H-Haloperidol
    E-Eritromycin
30. Asthma drugs: leukotriene inhibitor action
31. zAfirlukast: Antagonist of lipoxygenase
    zIlueton: Inhibitor of LT receptor
32. Beta blockers –BOBPA-
33. Betaxolol, oxprenolol, bisoprolol, propranolol, acebutolol, .
34. Beta blockers: B1 selective- MEAA- Acebutalol, Atenolol, Esmolol, Metoprolol.
    B1, B2 non-selective: PPT-Pindolol, Propanalol, Timolol.
35. Antirheumatic agents (disease modifying): CHAMP:
    C-Cyclophosphamide
    H-Hydroxycloroquine and choloroquinine
    A-Auranofin and other gold compounds
    M-Methotrexate
    P-Penicillamine
36. HMG-CoA reductase inhibitors (statins): side effects, contraindications, interactions HMG-CoA:
    Side effects:
    H-Hepatotoxicity
    M-Myositis [aka rhabdomyolysis]
    Contraindications:
    G-Girl during pregnancy/ Growing children
    · Interactions:
    C-Coumarin/ Cyclosporine
37. Serotonin syndrome: Causes- HARM:
    H-Hyperthermia
    A-Autonomic instability (delirium)
    R-Rigidity
    M-Myoclonus
38. Therapeutic index: formula TILE:
    TI = LD50 / ED50
39. Antiarrhythmics: class III members- BIAS:
    B-Bretylium
    I-Ibutilide
    A-Amiodarone
    S-Sotalol
40. MAOIs: indications MAOI'S:
    M-Melancholic [classic name for atypical depression]
    A-Anxiety
    O-Obesity disorders [anorexia, bulemia]
    I-Imagined illnesses [hypochondria]
    S-Social phobias

41. K+ increasing agents- K-BANK:
    K-K-sparing diuretic
    B-Beta blocker
    A-ACEI
    N-NSAID
    K-Ksupplement
42. Ribavirin: indications RIBAvirin:
    R-RSV
    I-Influenza B
    A-Arenaviruses (Lassa, Bolivian, etc.)
43. Syndrome of inappropriate antidiuretic hormone secretion(SIADH)-inducing drugs - ABCD:
    A-Analgesics: opioids, NSAIDs
    B-Barbiturates
    C-Cyclophosphamide/ Chlorpromazine/ Carbamazepine
    D-Diuretic (thiazide)
44. Diuretics: thiazides: indications "CHIC
    C-CHF
    H-Hypertension
    I-Insipidous
    C-Calcium calculi
45. Parkinsonism drugs- SALAD:
    S-Selegiline
    A-Anticholinenergics (trihexyphenidyl, benzhexol, ophenadrine)
    L-L-Dopa + peripheral decarboxylase inhibitor (carbidopa, benserazide)
    A-Amantadine
    D-Dopamine postsynaptic receptor agonists (bromocriptine, lisuride,pergolide)
46. Thrombolytic agents- USA:
    U-Urokinase
    S-Streptokinase
    A-Alteplase (tPA)
47. Morphine effects at mu receptor- PEAR:
    P-Physical dependence
    E-Euphoria
    A-Analgesia
    R-Respiratory depression
48. Morphine effects- MORPHINES:
    M-Miosis
    O-Orthostatic hypotension
    R-Respiratory depression
    P-Pain supression
    H-Histamine release/ Hormonal alterations
    I-Increased ICT
    N-Nausea
    E-Euphoria
    S-Sedation
49. Anticholinergic side effects - ABCD'S
    A-Anorexia
    B-Blurry vision

  C-Constipation/ Confusion
  D-Dry Mouth
  s-Sedation/ Stasis of urine
50. Antiarrhythmics: classification I to IV -MBA College
  M-Membrane stabilizers (class I)
  B-Beta blockers
  A-Action potential widening agents
  C-Calcium channel blockers
51. Teratogenic drugs -WETRATO:
  W-Warfarin
  E-Epileptic drugs: phenytoin, valproate, carbamazepine
52. T-Thalidomide
  R-Retinoid
  A-ACE inhibitor
  T-Third element: lithium
  O-OCP and other hormones (eg danazol)
53. Epilepsy types- FM PAW
  F-Focal
54. M-Myoclonic
  G-Grand mal
  P-Petit mal (absence)
55. A-Atonic
  W-West syndrome
  Drugs of choice- Triple V ACE
  V-Valproate
  V-Valproate
  VValproate
  A-ACTH
  C-Carbamazepine
  E-Ethosuximide
56. Pulmonary infiltrations inducing drugs "Go BAN Me!":
  Go-Gold
  B-Bleomycin/ Busulphan/ BCNU
  A-Amiodarone/ Acyclovir/ Azathioprine
  N-Nitrofurantoin
  M-Melphalan/ Methotrexate/ Methysergide
57. Respiratory depression inducing drugs "STOP
  S-Sedatives and hypnotics
  T-Trimethoprim
  O-Opiates
  P-Polymyxins
58. Benzodiazapines: safe to use in liver failure- LOT:
  L-Lorazepam
  O-Oxazepam
  T-Temazepam
59. TB: antibiotics used STRIPE:
  St-STreptomycin
  R-RIfampicin
  I-Isoniazid

P-Pyrizinamide
E-Ethambutol
60. Vigabatrin: mechanism - GABA-TRIN:
61. GABA Transferase Inhibition
62. Propythiouracil (PTU): mechanism - inhibits PTU:
P-Peroxidase/ Peripheral deiodination
T-Tyrosine iodination
U-Union (coupling)
63. Beta-blockers: nonselective beta-blockers "Tim Pinches His Nasal Problem"
Tim-Timolol
Pin-Pindolol
His-Hismolol
Na-Naldolol
Pro-Propranolol
64. Enoxaparin (prototype low molecular weight heparin): action, monitoring EnoXaprin only acts on factor Xa.
Monitor Xaconcentration, rather than APTT.
65. Nicotinic effects -MTWTF (days of week):
M-Mydriasis/ Muscle cramps
T-Tachycardia
W-Weakness
T-Twitching
H-Hypertension/ Hyperglycemia
F-Fasiculation
66. Muscarinic effects- SLUG BAM:
S-Salivation/ Secretions/ Sweating
L-Lacrimation
U-Urination
G-Gastrointestinal upset
B-Bradycardia/ Bronchoconstriction/ Bowel movement
A-Abdominal cramps/ Anorexia
M-Miosis
67. Hypertension treatment -ABCD:
ACE inhibitors/ AngII antagonists (Alpha agonists also)
B-Beta blockers
C-Calcium antagonists
D-Diuretics (sometimes vasoDilators also)
68. Phenytoin: adverse effects PHENYTOIN:
P-P-450 interactions
H-Hirsutism
E-Enlarged gums
N-Nystagmus
Y-Yellow-browning of skin
T-Teratogenicity
O-Osteomalacia
I-Interference with B12 metabolism (hence anemia)
N-Neuropathies: vertigo, ataxia, headache

69. Gynaecomastia-causing drugs DISCOS:
    D-Digoxin
    I-Isoniazid
    S-Spironolactone
    C-Cimetidine
    O-Oestrogens
    S-Stilboestrol
70. Amiodarone: action, side effects 6 P's:
    P-Prolongs action potential duration
    P-Photosensitivity
    P-Pigmentation of skin
    P-Peripheral neuropathy
    P-Pulmonary alveolitis and fibrosis
    P-Peripheral conversion of T4 to T3 is inhibited -> hypothyroiditis.
71. Beta blockers with intrinsic sympathomimetic activity-PC

    Pindolol and Carteolol have high and moderate ISA respectively,
    making them acceptable for use in some diabetics or asthmatics despite the fact that they are non-seletive beta blockers.
72. Physostigmine vs. Neostigmine- LMNOP:
    L-Lipid soluble
    M-Miotic
    N-Natural
    O-Orally absorbed well
    P-Physostigmine
    · Neostigmine, on the contrary, is:
    Water soluble
    Used in myesthenia gravis
    Synthetic
    Poor oral absorption
73. Monoamine oxidase inhibitors: "PIT
    P-Phenelzine
    I-Isocarboxazid
    T-Tranylcypromine
74. Antibiotics contraindicated during pregnancy MCAT:
    M-Metronidazole
    C-Chloramphenicol
    A-Aminoglycoside
    T-Tetracycline
75. Etoposide: action, indications, side effect "TOP":
    T-Testicular carcinoma
    O-Oat cell carcinoma of lung
    P-Prostate carcinoma
    · Side effect:
    Affects TOP of your head, causing alopecia
76. Antimuscarinics: members, action "Inhibits Parasympathetic And Sweat":
    I-Ipratropium
    P-Pirenzepine
    A-Atropine

S-Scopolamine
· Muscarinic receptors at all parasympathetic endings sweat glands in sympathetic.
77. Lithium: side effects LITHIUM:
L-Leukocytes Increased (leukocytosis)
T-Tremors
H-Hypothyroidism
I-Increased Urine
M-Moms beware (teratogenic)
78. Osmotic diuretics: GUM:
G-Glycerol
U-Urea
M-Mannitol
79. Narcotics side effects "SCRAM:
S-Synergistic CNS depression with other drugs
C-Constipation
R-Respiratory depression
A-Addiction
M-Miosis
80. Benzodiazepines: antidote "Benflu":
Benzodiazepine effects off with Flumazenil.
81. SSRIs: side effects SSRI:
S-Serotonin syndrome
S-Stimulate CNS
R-Reproductive disfunctions in male
I-Insomnia
82. Depression: 5 drugs causing - PROMS:
P-Propranolol
R-Reserpine
O-Oral contraceptives
M-Methyldopa
S-Steroids
83. Sex hormone drugs: male "Feminine Males Need Testosterone":
F-Fluoxymesterone
M-Methyltestosterone
N-Nandrolone
Testosterone
84. Ca++ channel blockers: uses CA MASH:
C-Cerebral vasospasm/ CHF
A-Angina
M-Migranes
A-Atrial flutter, fibrillation
S-Supraventricular tachycardia
H-Hypertension
85. Benzodiazepenes: drugs which decrease their metabolism-IOC:
I-Isoniazid
O-Oral contraceptive pills
C-Cimetidine

86. Warfarin: metabolism -SLOW:
    S-Small lipid-soluble molecule
    L-Liver: site of action
    O-Oral route of administration.
    W-Warfarin
87. Opioids effects -BAD AMERICANS:
    B-Bradycardia & hypotension
    A-Anorexia
    D-Diminished pupilary size
    A-Analgesics
    M-Miosis
    E-Euphoria
    R-Respiratory depression
    I-Increased smooth muscle activity (biliary tract constriction)
    C-Constipation
    A-Ameliorate cough reflex
    N-Nausea and vomiting
    S-Sedations
88. Tetracycline: teratogenicity TEtracycline is a
    TE-TEratogen that causes staining of
    TEeth in the newborn.
89. Myasthenia gravis: edrophonium vs. pyridostigmine eDrophonium
    is for Diagnosis.
    pyRIDostigmine is to get RIDof symptoms.
90. Narcotic antagonists The Narcotic Antagonists
    are NAloxone and NAltrexone.
    · Important clinically to treat narcotic overdose.
91. Inhalation anesthetics -SHINE:
    S-Sevoflurane
    H-Halothane
    I-Isoflurane
    N-Nitrous oxide
    E-Enflurane
92. Disulfiram-like reaction inducing drugs "PM PMT"
    P-Procarbazine
    M-Metronidazole
    PMT-Cefo (Perazone, Mandole, Tetan).
93. Delerium causing drugs- ACUTE CHANGE IN MS:
    A-Antibiotics (biaxin, penicillin, ciprofloxacin)
    C-Cardiac drugs (digoxin, lidocaine)
    U-Urinary incontinence drugs (anticholinergics)
    T-Theophylline
    E-Ethanol
    C-Corticosteroids
    H-H2 blockers
    A-Antiparkinsonian drugs
    N-Narcotics (esp. mepridine)
    G-Geriatric psychiatric drugs
    E-ENT drugs

I-Insomnia drugs
N-NSAIDs (eg indomethacin, naproxin)
M-Muscle relaxants
S-Seizure medicines

94. Direct sympathomimetic catecholamines -DINED:
D-Dopamine
I-Isoproterenol
N-Norepinephrine
E-Epinephrine
D-Dobutamine

95. Nitrofurantoin: major side effects- NFA:
N-Neuropathy (peripheral neuropathy)
F-Fibrosis (pulmonary fibrosis)
A-Anemia (hemolytic anemia)\

96. Methyldopa: side effects METHYLDOPA:
M-Mental retardation
E-Electrolyte imbalance
T-Tolerance
H-Headache/ Hepatotoxicity
psYcological upset
L-Lactation in female
D-Dry mouth
O-Oedema
P-Parkinsonism
A-Anaemia (haemolytic)

97. Steroids: side effects- BECLOMETHASONE:
B-Buffalo hump
E-Easy bruising
C-Cataracts
L-Larger appetite
O-Obesity
M-Moonface
E-Euphoria
T-Thin arms & legs
H-Hypertension/ Hyperglycaemia
A-Avascular necrosis of femoral head
S-Skin thinning
O-Osteoporosis
N-Negative nitrogen balance
E-Emotional liability

98. Sodium valproate: side effects- VALPROATE:
V-Vomiting
A-Alopecia
L-Liver toxicity
P-Pancreatitis/ Pancytopenia
R-Retention of fats (weight gain)
O-Oedema (peripheral oedema)
A-Appetite increase

    T-Tremor
    E-Enzyme inducer (liver)
99. Lithium: side effects- LITH:
    L-Leukocytosis
    I-Insipidus [diabetes insipidus, tied to polyuria]
    T-Tremor/ Teratogenesis
    H-Hypothyroidism.
100. Lead poisoning: presentation- ABCDEFG:
    A-Anemia
    B-Basophilic stripping
    C-Colicky pain
    D-Diarrhea
    E-Encephalopathy
    F-Foot drop
    G-Gum (lead line)
101. Beta-blockers: main contraindications, cautions -ABCDE:
    A-Asthma
    B-Block (heart block)
    C-COPD
    D-Diabetes mellitus
    E-Electrolyte (hyperkalemia)
102. Metabolism enzyme Inducers-RBC GPP
103. R-Rifampin
    B-Barbiturates
    C-Carbamazepine
    G-Grisoefulvin
    P-Phenytoin
    P-Phenobarb
104. Cholinergics (eg organophosphates): effects - LESS DUMB:
    L-Lacrimation
    E-Excitation of nicotinic synapses
    S-Salivation
    S-Sweating
    D-Diarrhea
    U-Urination
    M-Micturition
    B-Bronchoconstriction
105. Routes of entry: meds/toxins-Triple I A.
    Injection
    inhalation
    ingestion
    absorption
106. Hepatic necrosis: drugs causing-VAH:
    V-Valproic acid
    A-Acetaminophen
    H-Halothane
107. Bleomycin: action "Bleo-Mycin Blows
    My DNA to bits":

Bleomycin works by fragmenting DNA (blowing it to bits).
MyDNA signals that its used for cancer (targeting self cells).

108. Beta-1 vs Beta-2 receptor location "You have 1 heart and 2 lungs":
    Beta-1 are therefore primarily on heart.
    Beta-2 primarily on lungs.
109. Beta-blockers: side effects "BBC LIVR
    B-Bradycardia
    B-Bronchoconstriction
    C-Claudication
    L-Lipids-ve Inotropic action
    V-Vivid dreams & nightmares
    R-Reduced sensitivity to hypoglycaemia